LOCKED OUT

ELDER NEGLECT AND THE KEYS TO CHANGE

CANDACE E. ESHAM

Locked Out

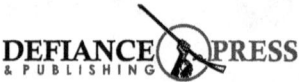

DEFIANCE **PRESS**
& PUBLISHING

ISBN-13: 978-1-966625-01-8 (Paperback)
ISBN-13: 978-1-966625-00-1 (eBook)

Published by Defiance Press & Publishing, LLC

Bulk orders of this book may be obtained by contacting Defiance Press & Publishing, LLC. www.defiancepress.com.

Public Relations Dept. – Defiance Press & Publishing, LLC
281-581-9300

Defiance Press & Publishing, LLC
281-581-9300
info@defiancepress.com

LOCKED OUT

ELDER NEGLECT AND THE KEYS TO CHANGE

CANDACE E. ESHAM

DEFIANCE PRESS
& PUBLISHING

Table of Contents

Part 1

Part 2

Part 3

Preface

"Life is good… hang on!" These were the last words my grandmother wrote before she died. Finding them months later gave me the strength to pursue an investigation into her neglect and advocate for others who suffer harm in long-term care facilities. My grandmother, whom I call Memom, wrote this sentence to her physician as she was suffering from a severe foot wound our family knew nothing about. The COVID-19 pandemic and resulting lockdowns kept us and many families of long-term care facility residents in the dark. Locking out families led to staff making key decisions regarding resident welfare absent family input, sometimes causing adverse outcomes, including neglect and death. These tragic losses occurred before the pandemic and will continue until systemic changes are implemented. The pandemic lockdowns only exacerbated an already broken long-term care system.

The grief one experiences after losing a loved one is not a single event or a process with stages to pass through, allowing one to get to the other side. Once a traumatic event happens in someone's life, their entire being changes. The big things and small things in life are all impacted by the loss. Missing relatives at lifetime events such as weddings and holidays hits hard, but so does not being able to call for simple conversations about a Phillies baseball game.

Memom lived her life to the fullest every day, and her family meant the world to her. A shining light who always saw the best in people, she never wanted to be a burden. Despite challenges throughout her life, she always persevered with joy and believed in doing something that made her happy each day. Faith was a preeminent and enduring value, and her love of God could be seen in her life's actions. Memom always put others first; my connection with her formed even before I was born due to the unexpected loss of my grandfather. Memom's legacy lives on in people who advocate for those who can't speak up for themselves. As a nurse who specialized in geriatric care, Memom was let down by the profession she dedicated her career to until she retired at age 68. Memom spent 17 years caring for residents of the Hospital for the Chronically Ill in Smyrna, Delaware, always prioritizing patient safety. Considered a "facility of last resort," it was a home for residents with no other options, and Memom treated each resident as though they were a family member.

After her retirement and following the death of her husband, Memom became a resident of an assisted living facility in Delaware, where she loved to play games, participate in all activities involving costumes, and carry on as the social butterfly she had always been. Capable of making her own life choices, we supported her decision to move into the facility and stay, even throughout the pandemic. She valued her independence and believed the accommodations at the assisted living facility were enough to help her continue an active lifestyle. Residents of the rural community Memom moved from did not have access to activities unless they had transportation. The assisted living facility provided transport to doctor's appointments and the local senior center for dances and other special events.

We believed Memom was enjoying her life at the assisted living facility, but after her death, we learned through her journal entries about what really happened when we weren't there. Never one to complain, Memom didn't mention how often no one would help her get dressed in the morning, how no one applied cream to her back when she had shingles—and how painful this was—or how lonely she was on days with few activities.

My Memom did not die of old age or its various complications; she died because medical professionals viewed her as old and, in a pandemic, not worthy of appropriate care. They failed to escalate her care as her foot wound worsened; they failed to give us vital information about the risks.

I struggle with how people who have dedicated their careers to helping others could look past her wounds and not escalate her case in order to provide her the proper treatments. Other significant health issues occurred before the lockdown; however, my mother and I discovered the injuries and ensured quality care was provided so Memom could heal. These injuries could have killed Memom had we not gotten involved.

On March 12, 2020, a state of emergency was declared by the Governor of Delaware, and long-term care facilities were locked up. No visitors were allowed, and residents were restricted to their rooms. For months, staff were the only people allowed in facilities, excluding normal oversight such as that from ombudsmen, state surveyors, and family members. The staff focused on controlling the spread of the virus, thinking that was the biggest threat to the safety of the residents. Every decision at the facility centered around preventing the spread of COVID, yet facility cases ran rampant. By January 2021, 39 of the 85 residents tested positive for COVID at one point, according to the State of Delaware, with four deaths due to the virus according to the state tracking website (https://news.delaware.gov/2021/01/16/delaware-surpasses-1000-total-deaths-related-to-covid-19-new-positive-cases-remain-elevated/). Meanwhile, other harm was crippling residents—and in Memom's case, that took her life.

My family only knows what happened during the lockdown from our outside experience and from medical records we received after Memom's death. We will never know what it was truly like for Memom since she was always supervised during the few visits we were allowed to have between March 2020 and her death in February 2021. We made no visits to Memom's room after the lockdown in March 2020; even window visits were monitored via the aide's phone on speaker. iPad devices and walkie-talkies provided by the facility were never charged and available for our use.

Since losing Memom, I have encountered countless families across the United States who grapple with the unknown truth about the neglect their loved ones suffered before dying in these facilities—before, during, and after the pandemic. Stories of how the loss and suffering have not only broken individuals but have completely broken families. Haunted by missing answers, they push for years for investigations, sometimes through lawsuits, to seek and obtain justice. Disagreements amongst siblings sometimes occur, where some never talk about the neglect again rather than continuing to battle for information. Family members blame themselves for what happened, replaying decisions made to keep their loved ones in an institution. Others developed health problems of their own due to the pain of loss. Neglect happened before the pandemic, during the pandemic, and it will continue to happen until the perception of the elderly changes in society and in systems charged with their care. Individual heartbreak and suffering are always behind the statistics and data on harm at these facilities. Unless people experience this tragedy, it is too easy for them to say "they had a good life" regarding those who've perished—and believe that should be enough to satisfy those left behind. It is simply too easy to minimize the ripple effect of that harm.

To honor Memom, I decided to dedicate my time, energy, and skills to advocate for our aging residents rather than holding onto my anger and grief about her passing and about the lack of action and policies that caused it. I began voicing the need for regulatory changes for elders in August 2020, concerned about the welfare of Memom. Public awareness of the systemic neglect of seniors in long-term care facilities did not occur until the local newspaper featured a series of investigative stories, including Memom's tragedy. In October 2023, I founded the Delaware Elder Care Advocacy Coalition. Our mission is to promote legislation for aging Delawareans to ensure they are able to thrive and receive quality medical care. Media coverage pressured state legislators to finally propose revisions to regulations related to long-term care. Across the United States, systemic changes are necessary in the way we provide care to seniors. Advocating for better care has illuminated the challenge of bringing about those changes. Powerful lobbyists, legislators fearful of facility closure threats, and the denial of widespread neglect provide obstacles to improving care. My expertise in performance improvement, advocacy, understanding regulations, and networking has led to progress in awareness and new legislation in the state of Delaware. Realizing this progress has helped me truly start healing. Progress in legislative changes, including a long-term care bill package and being active members of a state-level Caucus on Aging, earned my coalition the 2024 Delaware Lt. Governor's Challenge Community Spotlight Award. The United States Senate Special Committee on Aging met in January 2024 to discuss assisted living facilities for the first time in 20 years, acknowledging the urgency needed for changes to quality, transparency, and cost. According to testimony, "nearly a million Americans live in more than 30,000 assisted living facilities across our nation." By 2050, "nearly one in four Americans will be 65 or older."

Utilizing best practices, as well as learning challenges at a state and national level, helped me develop an advocacy plan. Sharing stories from other families across the country who have suffered losses due to neglect highlights the pervasiveness of harm to elders. It is my hope that those who read this book will understand the epidemic of neglect facing our aging residents. Further, I strive to be a source of inspiration for readers who will learn that a small, dedicated group of advocates with a focused mission can make a meaningful difference.

Part 1

Inside the Assisted Living Facility

Memom's Heart of Gold

Mary Claudia Jones Barthelmeh, my Memom, was born on July 9, 1924, on a sharecropper farm near Toccoa, Georgia. She was the first child of Claude and Lucilla Purcell. She often joked that her father was hoping she would be born on the Fourth of July, so this was the first, but not the only occasion, where she arrived late. She lost her own mother due to sepsis, a deadly infection, after the birth of her sister when she was just three years old. Memom was raised by her father and her beloved grandmother, who instilled in her faith, fortitude, and joyfulness. Her sister was raised in town by her aunt. Memom told me that her family was so poor, like so many other rural Georgia families, they didn't even realize there was a Great Depression. They had plenty of homegrown and canned food, cows for milk, hogs for canned pork or curing, and chickens from the barnyard for eggs and meat. Memom reminisced that her family was rich in that they had an abundance of food, warmth, and love.

After high school, Memom attended Toccoa Falls Institute through President Franklin D. Roosevelt's National Youth Administration program and worked for the college vice president. The woodworking shop was next door, and when the guys needed a Band-Aid, she would provide first aid. That was when she decided nursing was her calling. Going to the movies during World War II was a treat that helped American citizens escape the news of cruelty occurring throughout the world. In 1943, before one of the movies, Memom's interest was piqued by a trailer advertising free tuition at Emory University in Atlanta, Georgia. This offer was for students who signed up to be cadet nurses. She saw the need to serve her country and knew that paying for school would otherwise be impossible, so she left Toccoa, Georgia, in January 1944 to join the Cadet Nurse program at Emory University. Her aunts told her she would never make it and wouldn't take her to the train station, so she scheduled a taxi to pick her up at 6:30 a.m., and she never looked back. Whenever her college courses were challenging, her aunts' predictions motivated her to excel. Her final thesis on providing community-based care in rural areas is ironically an issue our country still struggles with today.

While taking classes at Emory University, she met Richard Barth, who would become her first husband. Memom and her best friend, Anne, enjoyed playing doubles tennis. One afternoon, Memom saw a men's doubles pair—Richard and his best friend—playing tennis. His friend bet him a dollar he could not get a date with her. Richard and Memom exchanged information about which dormitory they stayed in and began dating. A few months later, Richard gave Memom his fraternity pin as a symbol of engagement. Richard was in the Navy pre-med program at Emory University. They dated for more than a year before marrying in the campus chapel at Emory on August 22, 1946. Richard's tennis partner was his best man. After graduating, Richard was accepted into the Navy and enrolled in a medical program at Amherst College in Massachusetts.

Memom completed her practicum for pediatric nursing at Bellevue Hospital in New York City from January 1947 to July 1947. While there, she was recruited for modeling and was featured in a photo shoot but wanted to dedicate her career to nursing. After completing her practicum, she took a job at the Amherst College infirmary. Richard had Hodgkin's disease when he was 14 years old but had been in remission for many years. Sadly, the disease returned, and he died on May 8, 1948. Once Richard passed, Memom continued living with his parents and took a job at the Smith College infirmary.

Memom met my grandfather, Walt Jones, a World War II pilot, in Springfield, Massachusetts, at the Sheraton Hotel after she finished playing tennis nearby. Her friend Grace decided they should get dressed up and go to the Sheraton Hotel for a gimlet, a drink Memom read about in a novel. Memom and my grandfather talked outside the hotel briefly; then he asked for her number. Without a pen or paper, Memom wrote her number with lipstick on a napkin. On Labor Day weekend, they went to the beach with her friend Grace and his friend Lee. Less than a year later, on June 16, 1952, they married. They were deployed to Hawaii, where they spent a three-year honeymoon and returned to the states with a surprise for their parents – my mom, Lucilla. They moved to Dover, Delaware, in 1965. My grandfather served as the mortuary officer at the Dover Air Force Base after his career as a pilot ended. Walt and his dad built a house on Old Mill Road, where my grandparents would retire after deployment to Japan, San Francisco, and Illinois. Memom renewed her nursing license at age 50. She worked at the Hospital for the Chronically Ill in Smyrna, where she treated every patient with utmost care, compassion, and kindness until she retired at age 68. Sometimes, she was older than her residents. This facility, established in 1931, is a nursing facility for Delawareans with no income or no place to live. Most of the residents had no family to support or care for them, but Memom always ensured her patients felt loved. Celebrating holidays, anniversaries, and birthdays was as much a part of her nursing day as providing medical care to her patients. She never felt it a burden and made sure no one died alone. Memom cherished scrapbook photos of her patients and coworkers, and notes from staff expressing their gratitude for being able to work with her at the Hospital for the Chronically Ill. Memom's beautiful smile, selflessness, kindness, and positive outlook on life remain her legacy decades after her retirement.

As Memom's first grandchild, I had a special bond with her from the beginning. A month before I was born, my grandfather passed away after a quick battle with brain cancer. He was the love of Memom's life, and his death left a huge hole for her to fill. They did not even have the chance to enjoy retirement together before my grandfather lost his life. After I was born, my parents and I spent every other weekend in Dover, Delaware. Memom worked shifts at the Hospital for the Chronically Ill every other weekend. On the weekends she wasn't working, we loved taking beach trips and spending time together. I even lived with Memom for several months in my 20s while waiting for my house to be built in 2011. My favorite thing about Memom is that she made every day special. Even though I was in my twenties, she would pack my lunch each day with a folded napkin decorated with stickers and a note. In my bathroom, I display a sign she bought me stating, "Do one thing every day that makes you happy." Her passion and love for life were contagious.

Life at the assisted living facility before lockdown

Memom moved into the assisted living facility on July 1, 2014, after her late husband, Albert Barthelmeh, passed away. Living in a rural town in Delaware, she knew that as she aged, access to help for daily activities would be limited. There would be difficulty with things such as getting dressed, cooking meals, and taking showers. Prior to Memom moving, my mom researched reviews and complaints for each facility in the Dover area.

While Memom's husband was in hospice care dying from cancer, she toured an assisted living facility with good reviews and very few complaints. Since the facility was clean and close to her church, she made arrangements to move there. The only accommodations she needed at that time were assistance in getting dressed in the morning, help with meals in the dining hall, assistance with showers, and help with changing clothes for bed.

Memom loved being around people, playing games, and participating in social events. When she was growing up, Memom's father did not approve of games as they were associated with gambling, which was against their church's philosophy. After being raised in such a strict home with serious limits on fun, Memom relished the opportunity to play games of all sorts.

All activities at her assisted living facility were developed by the life enrichment coordinator. Not every assisted living facility has an employee in this role, as it is not mandated. Developing a program with activities for every interest takes skill; the coordinator at the assisted living facility, Kyla, set the bar high for expectations. Memom always loved Bingo and card games, Wii bowling, dressing up for any occasion, themed costume parties and special events, and interacting with others in the community. Seven days a week, Kyla scheduled various events including Bingo, pet therapy, reminiscing story time, visits from local school children, chair yoga, live music, and church services. Frequently, Memom won multiple games of Bingo in the same night along with the "cover-all," when all the numbers on her card were called.

Most events were held in the Bistro, a large, open room with chairs, tables, couches, and a jukebox with music from the 1940s, 1950s, and 1960s. The Bistro was also a popular gathering place for residents when activities weren't being held. Around holidays, Kyla designed events such as pumpkin decorating, an indoor Halloween Trick-or-Treat event for families, a Christmas party for residents and their relatives with live bands and appetizers, and a Fourth of July parade with classic cars. Family participation was always encouraged, and I attended special functions as often as I could. Our family rented the small dining room at Christmastime so Memom could host her family for Christmas lunch.

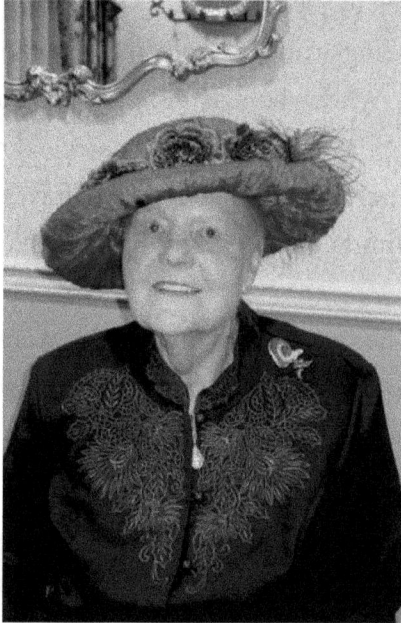

Memom at the "Taste of Derby" party

Memom never went more than two days in a row without having a visit from family or friends. She took a shuttle to her beloved Christ Episcopal Church every Sunday for worship and fellowship. My brother worked in Dover and would often stop for lunch in her dining hall. I tried to visit Memom every week, taking her to brunch, dinner, a pedicure, or a shopping trip. My mom loved to help Memom choose new outfits at Boscov's and go to Red Lobster for coconut shrimp or the Pub for a crabcake sandwich. An avid Phillies baseball fan, Memom carried the season schedule in her purse and never missed a game.

After Memom died, we brought home her red journals for each year in which she kept a detailed daily list of activities, including getting dressed, participating in events, and receiving visitors. If the Phillies were playing, she would describe the weather, game highlights, and the final score. While watching games with her in her room, we would cheer each run and grumble over bad calls loud enough for neighbors to hear us. I had the opportunity to treat her to box seats at Citizens Bank Park, the Phillies' stadium, twice while she was in the assisted living facility. She also documented nights when no one came to help her with a shower and how lonely she was at times.

Living in South Carolina from March 2017 through August 2018, I flew back every six weeks to see Memom. Carter, my Goldendoodle, came into our lives Memorial Day weekend 2018 and joined me on semi-weekly visits. Carter and Memom were very popular with the residents. Memom was voted resident ambassador. A canvas portrait of Memom and Carter graced the wall in the Bistro. Whenever Carter visited Memom, most of the residents asked if he could visit them too. Ann, who lived across the hallway, carried a Ziploc bag of bacon for Carter.

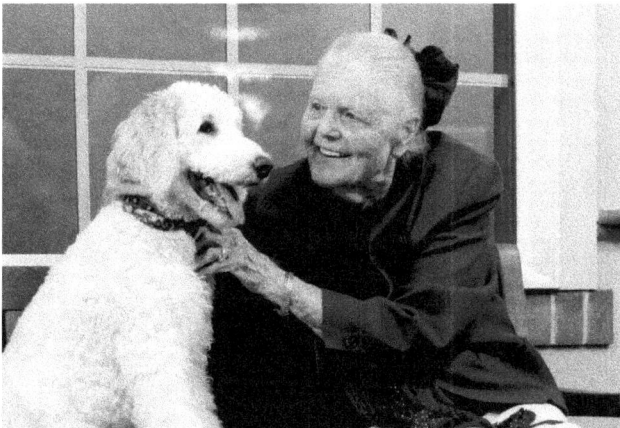

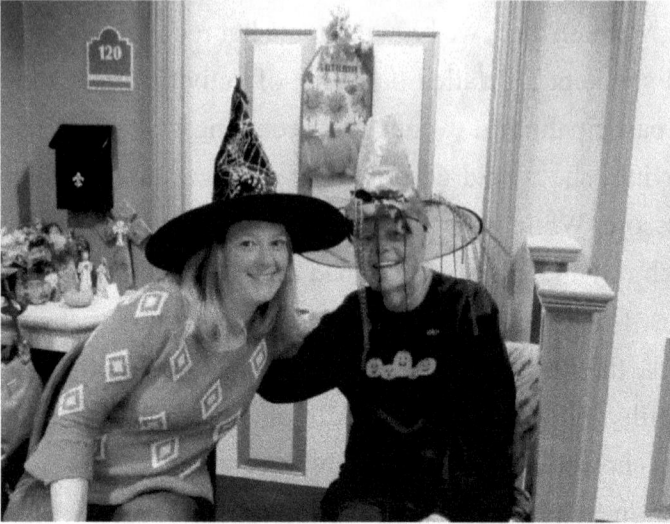

We believed Memom was happy living there; we believed our visits would help expose and solve any issues before they led to harm. One spring day in 2016, I stopped by to take Memom to lunch and to get a pedicure. When I got to her room, she mentioned her back feeling itchy and asked if I could look at it. Memom thought she accidentally used two laundry detergent pods, causing irritation to her skin. I lifted the back of her blouse and saw a rash of small, red blisters. Immediately, I knew this was not a reaction to soap powder; it was shingles. Assistance with showering was one of Memom's accommodations, and I wondered how anyone could miss such a distinct rash. Before we went to lunch, we walked down the hall to the nurse's station to report the shingles. Memom never complained and rarely asked for help. Reading her journals years later, I discovered several days when Memom requested that someone put calamine lotion on her back to ease the pain, but no one showed up. She barely slept those nights, restless due to the pain, but never told us.

Twice, Memom was admitted to the local hospital for urinary tract infections (UTIs). Dehydration can increase the risk of these infections, especially in older adults. According to the Cleveland Clinic, practicing proper genital-urinal hygiene and maintaining sufficient liquid intake can help promote urinary tract health in seniors. If there was enough staff at the facility, Memom received a shower twice a week; but this was not always the case. She did not get to choose which days she could shower. During her first ten months in the facility, her showers were scheduled on Tuesdays and Saturdays. Most weekends we would take Memom out to dinner or to my house or my parents' house for the evening. If she was not back by 7 p.m. Saturday evening, she missed her shower and would not have another opportunity to shower until the following Tuesday. Sometimes she would give herself a sponge bath, but that limited her ability to stay clean. When she requested to have her days of the week changed to accommodate her social schedule, a staff member came to her room demanding to know why she messed up their schedule. Memom detailed this interaction in her journal but never told us about the confrontation.

Each time she developed a UTI, Memom was taken by ambulance to the local hospital. Hallucinations and confusion were both signs she had a UTI. A family member drove to the hospital to ensure Memom had an advocate in the emergency room during both visits.

During one of the hospital stays, Memom developed hospital-acquired delirium. The combination of the infection and change in surroundings caused Memom to become very confused and agitated. Due to her behavioral change, the assisted living facility would not accept her once she was discharged from the hospital. Instead, she was sent to a rehabilitation facility where she was supposed to get physical therapy. When she arrived at the rehabilitation facility, a nurse was planning to give Memom Vicodin, a pain reliever, even though her file indicated she was allergic to this medication. My mom discovered the near miss, and we made sure a family member spent most of the day at the facility. We knew that with the lack of a private room and the noise levels at the facility, Memom would not get sufficient rest. Getting her back to her familiar assisted living environment would be imperative for her rest.

On a summer afternoon in August 2019, my mom had to take Memom to the dentist. The facility was supposed to provide transportation to appointments, but transportation was not a reliable amenity. When my mom arrived in the room to take her to the dentist, Memom was sitting in her recliner without her shoes on. Always so stylish, Memom loved to match her shoes with her outfit; she wanted Mom to find her purple flats. As my mom was putting on Memom's right shoe, Memom screamed out in pain. The outside of Memom's right foot was tender, red, and swollen. My mom reported the wound to the nurse but did not know the severity of it or realize the potential for the wound to become deadly.

Four days later, the nurse called 911 to have Memom taken to the local hospital. Streaks of red were rising from her foot up her calf. Diagnosed with cellulitis in her right leg and a stage 4 wound on the outside of her foot, Memom was admitted to the hospital and started on a strong antibiotic, Clindamycin. Cellulitis is a deep infection of the skin caused by bacteria. Wounds such as pressure injuries are classified into four stages. According to Johns Hopkins Medicine, with stage 4 wounds, "damage spreads to the muscle, bone, or joints. It can cause a serious bone infection called osteomyelitis. It can also lead to a possibly life-threatening blood infection called sepsis." Infections can cause confusion, and Memom suffered from confusion intermittently during the hospital stay. My aunt flew in from Colorado to provide relief for my mom, making sure someone was always in the hospital to advocate for Memom. Since Memom's mental status faded due to the infection, my mom or aunt could be present to speak with doctors about decisions regarding her care plan. In the middle of the night, a few days into the hospital stay, Memom told the doctor my mom and aunt had stolen all her money, and she asked that the police be alerted. Even though the doctor knew this wasn't true, they asked my mom and aunt to leave the room to try to calm Memom down. Memom never had a problem with memory, so it scared us to see her being so irrational. Eventually, the antibiotics controlled the infection, and Memom's clear thinking returned. After about a week in the hospital, she returned to the assisted living facility and had follow-up appointments with her podiatrist. Prior to these three admissions to the hospital, Memom was only in the hospital overnight when she gave birth to her three children.

A few days after she was settled back into the assisted living facility, an investigator from the Office of Long-term Care Residents Protection in the Division of Health Care Quality stopped by to see Memom. My mom and I never found out if the facility self-reported Memom's foot wound to the investigator or if another family member called the state department. Assisted living facility regulations list certain reportable incidents. This injury could have been included as a "serious, unusual, and/or life-threatening injury." The facilities are not licensed to take care of residents with stage 3 or stage 4 wounds. Staff was supposed to have training to identify when wounds exceed the level of care they could provide.

The investigator assigned had retired as a New York State police officer, moved to Delaware, and decided on a second career protecting elders against neglect. He interviewed Memom about her wound and her experience in the facility. In Memom's career as a geriatric nurse, she had to report coworkers for harming residents at the facility several times. Once, a resident contacted management about a nurse verbally mistreating them, and Memom discovered the nurse also retaliated when they heard about the complaint. I admired Memom for her moral compass and for always putting her patients first. She did not want to pursue an investigation into her foot wound. The investigator left her with his business card and offered to talk to her any time if she needed help in the future. Memom kept his card in her wallet; we found it after she passed. My mom and I believe she feared retaliation, and she did not want to leave her friends. The investigator also interviewed my mom. I remember us discussing the pros and cons of moving forward with the investigation.

My mom decided to tour a facility closer to her house—an hour away from Memom's current location—to see if we should move Memom. The facility sparkled and had a large chandelier in the entryway. A baby grand piano was in the sitting area, and the couches looked new. One thing stood out during the visit, however. During the middle of the afternoon, Mom saw no residents. All residents were sitting in their rooms; no one was participating in activities around the campus. Often called "the Chandelier effect," the meticulous landscaping outside and beautiful fixtures inside a facility are often what draws families in. While cleanliness is of paramount importance, a lack of activities for residents on a normal weekday is never a good sign. During Mom's visit, this was alarming.

After touring another facility, my mom and I decided we did not want to pursue an investigation. If we kept a closer eye on Memom, we were sure she would be safe. At the time, we didn't understand the danger of not demanding corrective actions to prevent another wound. For $7,000 out of pocket a month, we questioned what kind of care Memom was really getting. Also, later, I would wonder how many other families decided not to investigate neglect in fear of retaliation.

March 2020

When my mother visited on March 12, 2020—the day the first State of Emergency was declared by the Governor—she told me she had a feeling it would be the last time she would sit on my Memom's couch. This premonition turned out to be true, but we could not have expected the suffering Memom went through before she passed away on February 16, 2021. Across Delaware and across the country, assisted living facilities isolated family members from their loved ones while eliminating audits and classifying ombudsmen as "non-essential." The cumulative effect of these actions left the door open to neglect, suffering, and mental trauma. The pandemic only exacerbated the systemic issues festering for years in these long-term care facilities. We had our scares with injuries to Memom prior to the pandemic, but we'd always been able to alert the nurse at the facility since we were there so often.

The United States was originally told by President Trump that we would be locked down for two weeks and we would isolate in an attempt to "stop the spread" of COVID. Each state governor was given the authority to manage the public health emergency. I watched the news every day for updates on what was going on across the country and for information about deaths in long-term care facilities. The death rate across those facilities was alarming. Governors of New York, New Jersey, Pennsylvania, and Michigan issued orders for residents sent to the hospital positive with COVID to be readmitted to long-term care facilities even if they were still positive. Specifically, on March 25, 2020, the New York Governor ordered, "No resident shall be denied re-admission or admission to [a nursing home] solely based on a confirmed or suspected diagnosis of COVID-19. [Nursing homes] are prohibited from requiring a hospitalized resident who is determined medically stable to be tested for COVID-19 prior to admission or readmission."

On August 26, 2020, the Department of Justice initiated an investigation under the Civil Rights of Institutionalized Persons Act into the decisions made by these state governors. The investigation stated:

"According to the Centers for Disease Control, New York has the highest number of COVID-19 deaths in the United States, with 32,592 victims, many of them elderly. New York's death rate by population is the second highest in the country with 1,680 deaths per million people. New Jersey's death rate by population is 1,733 deaths per million people—the highest in the nation. In contrast, Texas' death rate by population is 380 deaths per million people; and Texas has just over 11,000 deaths, though its population is 50 percent larger than New York and has many more recorded cases of COVID-19—577,537 cases in Texas versus 430,885 cases in New York. Florida's COVID-19 death rate is 480 deaths per million; with total deaths of 10,325 and a population slightly larger than New York."

Texas and Florida did not force long-term care facilities to accept residents who were still positive for COVID. In fact, both states approved legislation allowing residents to choose an essential caregiver who may not be denied in-person visitation under most circumstances. Unfortunately, in July 2021, the Department of Justice called off the investigation. There was no clear reason for canceling it. A bipartisan, bicameral Essential Caregivers Act (H.R. 8331 and S. 4280) was introduced by U.S. Senators and U.S. Representatives in Connecticut, Texas, and New York in May 2024 in an attempt to protect residents nationwide from essential caregiver visitations. As of December 2024, the bill has not received enough votes to become law but has had equal support from both the Republican and Democratic parties. In the bill, it is estimated that 1,300,000 individuals resided in nursing homes in 2020 at the start of the pandemic, according to the National Center for Health Statistics of the Centers for Disease Control and Prevention.

This does not include residents of assisted living facilities, who were also isolated, as those facilities are regulated by the states. Significant harm was documented in the research for the bill, justifying the need to never isolate caregivers again. "During the pandemic, pressure ulcers in nursing home residents rose by 31 percent, the number of residents experiencing significant weight loss rose by 49 percent, the number of residents reporting feeling down, depressed, or hopeless rose by 40 percent, and the number of residents prescribed antipsychotic medications rose by 77.5 percent," according to the National Consumer Voice for Quality Long-Term Care. Premature deaths from "failure to thrive" in isolation were not uncommon.

The news coverage of the death rate in facilities in New York made me terrified for Memom's life. Two weeks of lockdowns morphed into months. We were told to keep isolated; we were not allowed to see family members in the hospital or long-term care facilities. Even as a manufacturing engineer, I was told to work remotely rather than in the office. While Delaware never mandated that facilities accept COVID-positive residents, I feared how government decisions could mean life or death for the elderly. Delaware Governor John Carney still had an active Public Health Emergency declared until the end of the day on May 11, 2023, resulting in over three years of free rein for executive order power by the Governor. Included in this order of power was for the Public Health Authority to be authorized to "direct vaccination, treatment, isolation, quarantine and such other measures as may be necessary to prevent or contain the spread of COVID-19" (reference link to public health emergency letter).

During the Public Health Emergency, staffing ratios and audits of facilities were not required. In fact, Eagles Law, which was established in Delaware in 2000 to dictate staffing ratios in skilled nursing home facilities, was waived through July 2024, well after the Public Health

Emergency ended. Even the waiver process, which is also a part of the law and is designed to show how residents and staff will be kept safe during the interim staffing issue, is not required. I did not know at the time how few regulations existed for assisted living facilities, including no staffing ratio requirements. Those were only established for skilled nursing facilities. The already substandard rules to protect patients and residents at long-term care facilities were not enforced to allow staff and facilities to focus on the Public Health Emergency. The Centers for Medicare & Medicaid Services requires skilled nursing facilities to be surveyed annually, with a grace period extending to every 15 months. There was no required frequency for assisted living facility surveys other than "regular." Delaware frequently does not follow these guidelines. Allowing facilities to go so long without being audited or provided with the appropriate levels of staff left our most vulnerable population open to neglect and harm.

Humans are not meant to live in isolation. History has shown that separating families and individuals can cause severe depression and other health issues. Medical professionals at Memom's assisted living facility saw enforcing the isolation as their duty and saw "protecting" Memom and others within the facility from COVID as their primary mission. Before the lockdown, a podiatrist would come to the facility once a month for routine resident foot examinations. This medical service was stopped for fear of an outside medical professional introducing the virus to residents and staff. My weekly trips to take Memom out to dinner or get a pedicure stopped, leaving me worried about her physical and mental safety. She had a cell phone but did not have the capability to video chat with any family. We were allowed to look through her window, which was often covered in dust, but we were not able to see her any other way. The virus and "containment of it" remained the primary focus for the staff despite them not being able to prevent outbreaks.

The first sign in lockdown

I vividly remember waking up to several text messages and missed calls from my mom on the morning of August 26, 2020. Memom had fallen in her room at 1:30 a.m. and was severely injured. When I returned Mom's call, she didn't have details but knew Memom's injuries were significant. At the time, we were also not aware of how lucky we were that the ambulance came for Memom. The assisted living facility provided each resident with a fall alert button necklace that, when activated, would call the main nurse station. Memom had purchased a Life Alert button before becoming a resident of the assisted living facility and wanted to keep that active for an extra sense of security. The night she fell, both buttons activated. No one at the assisted living facility answered the alert sent by the device they provided. The device Memom paid for called a center in New Jersey. When the call center operator wasn't able to get anyone to answer the phone at the facility, they tried to contact my uncle—the primary contact; he didn't pick up the phone. The alert called 911, and the ambulance showed up at the facility. The paramedics also tried to call, and no one at the assisted living facility answered the phone, so they started banging on the door. A staff member eventually came to the door to let the paramedics in. They found Memom face down fully dressed in street clothes. Every day, even during the pandemic, Memom dressed up in a pair of slacks, a shell top, and a beautiful jacket. The night before, no one had helped her get into her pajamas, one of the few accommodations she required. I knew she was in her dress clothes because I picked up her belongings at the hospital.

She was transported to the local hospital, Kent General Hospital, which is about 15 minutes from the assisted living facility. My mother received a phone call from the hospitalist, a physician working solely in the hospital setting, asking if Memom was "worth saving" due to her age. Still unclear on the severity of the injuries Memom had sustained, my mom questioned what the hospitalist meant by that. The hospitalist clarified that Memom would need to be transported to Christiana Hospital, the only Level 1 Trauma Center in the state of Delaware where a medical team could help her. The fall caused her to hit her head and lacerate her spleen; her head required 19 staples. Memom's advanced directive, a legal document specifying the kind of care to be given if one can't communicate, was on file at Kent General as that hospital was closest to her assisted living facility. The advanced directive specified Memom as "full code," meaning all medical treatments should be used to save her life. She was transferred via a helicopter ride of approximately 15 minutes due to her critical condition. The operation for repairing her spleen could not be performed at Kent General Hospital; the plan was to have the surgery at Christiana Hospital.

I went to the Christiana Emergency Room (ER) to meet her and get her settled into the surgical unit. This was the greatest amount of time I spent with her during the entire pandemic. I was and still am so thankful she was awake and knew what was going on, so I could spend time with her. When I first saw her, she didn't recognize me with a mask on, so I removed it. I held her hand and gave her hugs—the first she had received in months due to isolation requirements. Using my phone, I showed her pictures of Carter, my Goldendoodle, and tried to hide my fear and sadness. I had not seen her since March, and I was shocked at how much she had changed in even a few short months. Memom had never aged in my mind, but this injury made me realize how much the isolation had changed her. She even told me that if I had other things to do, I did not need to sit around and wait with her. Always focused on the bright side of life, she minimized her injuries and told me how exciting the helicopter ride was from Dover to Newark. She described the ride as smooth and couldn't believe she finally had the opportunity to ride in a helicopter. Memom always knew how to make the best of any situation, even when I knew she had to be in pain from her injuries.

A nurse came into the emergency room bay and told us Memom was ready to go up to the surgical waiting rooms. He let me ride in the back of the hospital patient transport elevator with them so I could spend more time with Memom. Once we got to the room, the nurse asked me to go to the waiting room while the staff transferred her into the bed and made her comfortable. I waited about 30 minutes in the family waiting room before being called back into Memom's room. Memom didn't have her hearing aids in her ears, so I explained to the nurse that Memom was sound of mind but just couldn't hear. Clarifying hearing issues is important to prevent staff from assuming an older person has cognitive issues.

Shortly after Memom settled into her room, a nurse led me to her room so I could spend more time with her. In the hallway on the way to her room, I told the nurse in the surgical unit that I knew Memom would be okay if she asked for her lipstick. He laughed and asked for more details. Memom had only been admitted to the hospital twice before: once for a urinary tract infection (UTI) and once for a wound from her shoes. Every other time she had been in the hospital, a family member met her there to ensure she had an advocate. Memom fully believed that if she dressed up and looked nice, the doctor would release her sooner. Since she was limited to a hospital gown until she was released, red lipstick was her go-to (Clinique or Maybelline). When I walked into the room, she immediately asked if I had lipstick. Feeling a sense of relief, I stayed with Memom for half an hour talking about the Phillies and their playoff possibilities. The nurse told me they would monitor Memom's vitals and relay the plan for surgery to us. Once I left the hospital, I would not be allowed to visit again due to COVID policies. Staff updated my mom each day with promising news about Memom's condition. She miraculously healed without surgery and returned to her assisted living facility on September 3, 2020. Her fall was entered in the state complaint system since falls resulting in any injury are required to be reported; however, we never received information about the investigation.

My mom visited Memom the week after she was released from the hospital and returned to the assisted living facility. Families were allowed 30-minute supervised porch visits when they weren't in their two-week lockdowns. Mom had an appointment on the porch; my grandmother was running late since she was in the bathroom. Because of the injuries she sustained from the fall, it was taking her more time than usual to move around the bathroom and the assisted living facility. Memom arrived late to the porch, and the front desk attendant came outside and said, "You have 12 minutes for your visit." There was no one waiting to use the porch—and my mother had driven over an hour to get there. My mother said she expected a full 30 minutes with Memom. With no scientific justification behind the "30-minute rule," it is truly disturbing how someone can enforce a rule that clearly impacted Memom's mental health. Obviously, there was no health reason to limit the already restrictive visit, so this felt punitive and controlling. An attendant was mandatory for each family visit, which meant no resident privacy.

My mom drove from Millsboro to Dover, a little over one hour each way, once a week to see Memom. On weeks when she wasn't allowed on the porch, she would visit through the window; luckily, Memom lived on the first floor. I felt guilty for not standing outside the window for a visit, but I could not handle the hurt of seeing her on the other side of the glass. Memom paid an extra $2,000 a month for an aide. Mom would coordinate when the aide was available to use her personal cell phone to communicate with my grandmother. The battery-powered walkie-talkies the facility provided for communication with families did not work. I had a hard time making visits work since I worked full time during the day and her aide was off on Saturdays. We had a ViewClix video box in her room so we could see her, but Memom usually didn't say much on there since it was hard for her to hear the monitor. This was how I noticed her room was dark during the day. A chair sat in front of her window; this blocked her ability to reach the pull cord for the blinds. If no one came into her room each morning to open the blinds, she sat in the dark, alone.

The second sign

In October 2020, I called the nurse and asked about visiting; she told me, "The governor is not allowing visitations." Hearing from friends who worked in healthcare in Kent County revealed a discrepancy between what we were being told by the staff at Memom's assisted living facility and what they were told at their facilities. I called the Delaware COVID Hotline to try to understand the criteria on visitation. I left a voicemail requesting information about how to know the status of restrictions on visitors in long-term care facilities in Kent County. Four weeks later, I received a call back. The phone representative told me that facilities would blame the state, but the state was allowing visitation at that time, particularly outdoor visits. She told me private facilities can require further restrictions, so I should refer to the corporate policy. On November 10, 2020, my mom emailed me a link to the corporate policy in place regarding visitation. The policy mandated a 14-day isolation for a confirmed positive COVID case with a requirement to test residents once a positive case occurs. However, the policy did not state to isolate each resident with a negative COVID test. With the corporate policy not aligning with the actions the facility staff took each week, I decided to investigate further. I called the corporate complaint hotline for the facility and was called back by the Regional Director of Care Services on November 18, 2020. I told him my concerns about not being able to see Memom. He said they were not restricting visitation and that they followed what the state was doing. He confirmed I should be able to visit, and I made an appointment to see her the next afternoon. At this point, I realized that the individual staff at the assisted living facility were coming up with their own rules without consulting the corporate director of nursing. Looking back, I realize that this incident was the second violation of my trust in the staff at the assisted living facility—the first being their lack of response to my call when she fell in August.

On Tuesday, November 19th, I drove about 45 minutes from my house in Middletown to Dover to have my first visit with Memom since I saw her in the hospital in August. It was supposed to be an outdoor porch visit, but since it was after my workday and the temperatures were in the 40s, they decided to shift the visit indoors. When I got to the facility entrance, I walked through the double doors to check in. I was told to go back through the doors and change out my face mask for their approved mask. Once I swapped out the mask as required, I signed in, recorded my temperature, and walked into the Bistro—the community gathering room to the right of the entrance. Only Memom sat in the Bistro, in a wheelchair with her mask on. I did not expect this to be a visit where we were supervised by three people. They stood outside of the room, but the doors were open. The supervision was to make sure I stayed in my chair, which was inside a square of blue tape. At this time, "social distancing," a measure of 6 feet between two people, was enforced, and physical contact was off-limits. I brought Memom some candy from my local candy shop and asked if I would be allowed to pass it across the table. While I was talking with Memom, the employees who were watching through the doorway would chime in to our conversation, which made me think about limiting what I said. As I was sitting in the room, I heard the front desk phone ring repeatedly, and the front desk attendant told many people that "we are not allowing visitors at this time," even though I knew it wasn't true because I had just spoken with the director. Since this was Thanksgiving week, I knew families especially wanted to spend time with their loved ones. This was the first major holiday when families were separated. I heard the receptionist say that video visits may be possible but not guaranteed due to how busy the staff was.

Memom didn't say much during the visit, and when I looked into her eyes, I could see fear and confusion. She had a hard time hearing me since my voice was muffled, and she couldn't see my mouth move. I was so overcome with emotions that it was hard for me to make small talk or act like this was a normal visit. It was the first time in my life that I had seen Memom and not been able to give her a hug. Even when I met her in the emergency room in August, I pulled my mask down to show her who I was and gave her a hug. It seemed like a nightmare to have to share small talk about my week when she was basically held hostage by the draconian policies. The visit felt both like slow motion—which I spent a lot of time holding back tears while thinking of something meaningful to say—and like the fastest 38 minutes of my life. I knew it was 38 minutes because the receptionist came over to the table to tell me they gave me an extra 8 minutes of visiting time. I didn't say anything to the regional nursing director about the conversations I overheard for fear of retaliation.

I planned on visiting weekly after that, even if it meant taking time off from work, and took off the week after Thanksgiving. I had a porch visit scheduled on December 1, 2020. When my mother and I showed up, we were confronted on the porch by two staff members and the director. A nurse handed me an email explaining the state mandate for no visitors and told me, "If I didn't like it, I could take her out of there." They told me they had heard that I reported their visitation restrictions to the regional nursing director via the corporate complaint hotline. They laughed as they asked how he was going to enforce anything. Then they screamed at me, "How do we know that you're safe and don't have COVID?" They followed that up by asking what my profession was, insinuating that I might get someone sick. They said they had not had a COVID outbreak and implied that my wanting to see Memom was putting people's lives at risk. During the confrontation with the staff, I brought up seeing Memom sitting in the dark during the day multiple times when I would call on the ViewClix video device. Memom always loved to get dressed up, put on her makeup, and be active during the day. She never wanted to sit in the dark, restricted to a recliner.

During our discussion, various people were going in and out of the facility with bandanas and other face coverings that were not the "approved" mask I was forced to wear the week before. After I asked the director why Memom's blinds would be shut and the room dark when I called on the ViewClix, she said, "Your grandmother wouldn't benefit from mental health help." Finally, the staff said they would make an exception and let us have a porch visit. I didn't ask for an exception, but I did think it was cruel to get her to the door, see us standing there, and have them tell her that she couldn't see us. My grandmother was sitting just inside the double doors to the entrance in a wheelchair in her socks. (We later realized she couldn't wear shoes due to her foot wound). Memom was excited for our visit but became visibly distressed when she overheard the confrontation. We were able to have a 30-minute supervised visit on the porch after her aide dressed her in a proper coat and blanket for the chilly 45-degree weather. I asked her aide why so many people were going in and out of the facility; she told me that it was COVID testing day for the staff members. Instead of staff going to a testing center, they conducted the COVID tests inside the facility in the private dining room. This meant that anyone going in could be positive for COVID, walking right past my Memom.

Impacts of Isolation

We had no idea how crushing the isolation from family and friends and most human contact was to Memom. I was mostly alone for 42 days during the beginning of the pandemic, only seeing people walking outside when I would take my dog for a walk. I kept my dog walker even though I was working from home since most of her clients stopped services. The ten minutes I would see her each day during the week truly were my main connection to humans. FaceTime and electronic forms of talking can only fulfill so much of that need to feel connected. However, unlike Memom, I could at least drive where I wanted and leave my room. Knowing how lonely and isolated I felt, I can't even imagine how Memom was feeling. She truly was the strongest person I have ever known. But no human is strong enough to thrive during a lockdown. Based on the health records we received after her death, there were definite signs of the isolation impacting her health.

On July 30, 2020, Memom was seen by an external agency for "increased anxiety and not sleeping well." Mom, the medical power of attorney, was not notified. There is only documentation of my uncle being contacted about labs being ordered. It is unclear what accommodations or follow-up would be provided based on the notes. On August 4, 2020, at around 9 p.m., the nurse documented the following:

"Resident in apartment states 'the people are coming to change their shoes through her window.' While walking through the apartment, myself and her reflection were in the window. Resident stated she could not go to bed while the people were there. Blinds were closed and the resident was reassured that I would help the people so she could rest. She felt better, she reported, watched baseball, and was reported to be sleeping in her bed. Power of attorney (POA) notified of incident. PCP (primary care physician) notified." My mom wasn't called, so we never knew who the facility nurse actually called.

On August 13, 2020, Memom was seen by an external nursing agency for follow-up from the labs and "seeing people in the apartment." The labs were normal, and they documented she was "sleeping better in bed and blinds closed earlier." They left a message for my uncle. Based on the notes, their solution to her anxiety was to simply close the blinds earlier in the evening. There was no plan discussed with the family or discussions about mental health care. According to the records, it's clear that her mental status was changing, which likely was impacting her sleep. One day in the early fall of 2020, I called on the ViewClix video chat to see how Memom was doing and noticed how dark the room was. She was sleeping in her recliner, which was unlike her before the isolation started. She may have taken a brief nap here and there but was usually out and about with activities. I called the nursing station after seeing the dark room; the nurse mentioned they decided to open the blinds in Memom's room "based on how she is doing that day." At the time, I didn't know how to respond since I didn't think speaking up would make a difference. The nurse seemed convinced that they were doing the right thing. When Mom and I had our visit after Thanksgiving, the nurse confronted us on the front porch of the facility. She stated she had heard we called to complain to the regional nursing director. The facility director told me that Memom wouldn't benefit from mental health services or treatment and that is why they decided to close the blinds.

Sadly, this is not the only knowledge I had of isolation taking its toll on residents in long-term care facilities. My best friend's grandmother lives in a facility in another state. Every day, her grandmother would go for walks and enjoy her independence. One day, she tested positive for COVID-19. She had no symptoms, but it was facility policy to remove the resident from their room and isolate them in another section of the facility. The room in a different part of the facility didn't even have its own telephone, and she lost track of the time of day without a clock. The nurse would have to bring a phone to the room if her grandmother wanted to speak with any family members. Even the window was nailed shut to prevent anyone from opening it.

Around 8 p.m. on August 18, 2020, Memom was found sitting on the bathroom floor in her apartment when a staff member arrived in her room after being paged. The residents of the facility wore a necklace with a button to alert staff when they fell or needed assistance. Memom's back was against the wall, and her walker was within reach. She did not state she was in any pain or discomfort at the time. A staff member called a family member to notify them of the fall.

The next time she fell was in the middle of the night from August 25th to August 26th. This time, the pendant she wore from the facility either did not alert the staff or the staff did not respond to the page. Luckily, Memom wore her own lifeline pendant that alerted an external facility, whose representative then called 911 when no one at Memom's facility answered. When I met Memom at the hospital, her bag of belongings included dress clothes, making me question why she wasn't in pajamas since she fell in the middle of the night. I began to worry about her sleep schedule and how that impacted her mental state. The next documentation of increased sleepiness and agitation was on October 14th. Still, there was no plan for how to handle the concern. The nurse simply documented the status, called the POA, and moved on with her day. I started calling on the ViewClix video chat device and noticed Memom's room was dark during the day due to the blinds being closed.

Florida government officials realized the harm in locking out families, and on September 1, 2020, Governor DeSantis allowed some visitation to residents of long-term care facilities as specified in the Division of Emergency Management Order Number 20-009. The order specified that visitors wear personal protective equipment (PPE), including a face mask, but allowed general visitors for all residents. Florida long-term care facilities did not see an increase in COVID-positive cases as a result of visitation, and residents of facilities were reunited with their loved ones. On April 6, 2022, Governor DeSantis signed Senate Bill 988, *No Patient Left Alone Act*, which guarantees families the right to visit their loved ones in hospitals, hospices, and long-term care facilities. Recognizing visitation as a fundamental right, Governor DeSantis stated in a press release, "Throughout the pandemic, the federal government has waived protections for families to visit their loved ones in hospitals and long-term care facilities. That is unacceptable. Here in Florida, we recognize that family and human connection is one of the most important aspects of physical, mental, and emotional well-being, and we are ensuring Floridians are never again denied the right to see their relatives and friends while in hospitals or nursing homes." Florida Representative Jason Shoaf claimed, "COVID showed us that while a virus can be deadly, depression and loneliness can be just as deadly. We all have heard and experienced the heart-wrenching stories of those in facilities cut off from their loved ones. This law will be a large step toward preventing this problem." I am glad I decided to hug Memom in August when she was in the hospital. Life is full of risks and decisions. If we don't look at the failures and admit them, how will we learn? Unfortunately, Delaware law did not change, and there are no protections for resident visitation rights if there are future public health emergencies as of December 2024.

Christmas

When I think of Christmas, I always think of Memom in a beautiful red suit with a dressy scarf, a sparkly pin, and a big red hair bow. She loved dressing up for holidays—really every day since she felt each day was a blessing. Each December, the assisted living facility would host a family party for the residents and two guests. It was my favorite event of the year at the facility. The activities coordinator would design a special menu of appetizers and have live music. Every table featured name tags so that families and residents with no family could celebrate Christmas together. Each year, Memom and I took a picture beside the giant tree in the foyer with her in a different red suit. One year, I got there early and saw Ann, her neighbor across the hall, milling around in the Bistro. She was scanning to see who was sitting with whom, then rearranging her family's name tags. I asked her why she was moving things around, and she said, "Life is too short to sit with boring people at dinner." I loved all Memom's friends at the facility and appreciated their unique personalities.

In December 2019, I had a pretty bad chest cold and debated with myself about whether or not I should go to the family party at the facility. I never wanted to take any illness into the facility, as everyone there was so susceptible to getting sick. I reasoned with myself that if I could take enough cold syrup not to cough and felt better the day of the event, then I would still go to the annual family Christmas party. At the time, I had no idea that it would be my last Christmas event and last picture with Memom. When I look at that picture, I think of how precious time is and that time is the greatest gift you can give someone.

Fast forward to December 2020: I talked to my mom about having a bad feeling the week after Thanksgiving when we had the outdoor visit. Other states, like West Virginia, had started giving the COVID

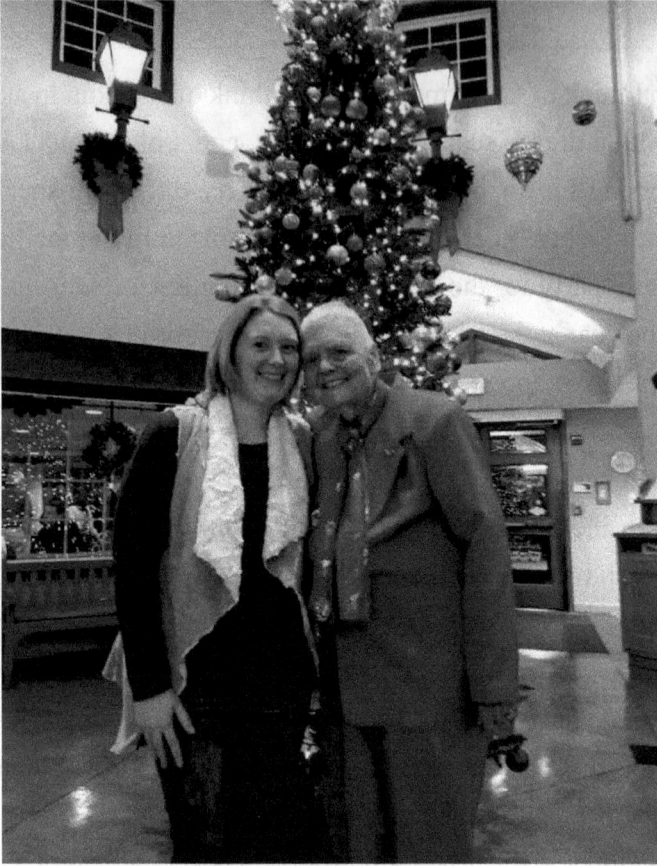

vaccine to residents in assisted living facilities and nursing homes to make sure the most vulnerable were protected. There are debates now as to how effective the vaccines are, but at the time, it seemed like the best way to protect the elderly. Also, in states where lockdowns were still in place, facilities providing the vaccine were easing restrictions and allowing residents to get back to their routines. I was researching states that were prioritizing getting the vaccine to the vulnerable over healthy healthcare workers and decided to write to anyone I thought could influence the state priorities in Delaware. I even started to attend my local representative's town halls. In these meetings, I shared the status of other states and came prepared to provide statistics or any data to support my case. With the holidays coming and no scheduled vaccine date for Memom, I begged my mom to talk with her brother and sister about bringing Memom to my parents' house for the holidays. The facility was on lockdown continuously after Thanksgiving, and I began to panic about not seeing Memom. Mom would go to the window of Memom's room and call her health aide's cell phone to see Memom while talking. The window had a screen and was covered in dust on the outside, but they could still see each other. With each passing week, we could see the strain of isolation, even though Memom seemed to always keep hope.

On the morning of December 23, 2020, my mom wrote an email to the Delaware State Department of Health begging for help to get Memom the vaccine.

Email:

I am writing on behalf of my 96 year old mother, Claudia Barthelmeh.
She is a resident of an assisted living facility.

She has been isolated from family and friends since March 12 and her health is degrading.

Now we have been informed that there are positive COVID-19 cases among the residents.

When can she receive the vaccine?

I am imploring you to help.

Lucilla Esham

We had no timeline for vaccine distribution from the facility or state officials. The combination of the virus raging through the facility, Memom's lack of human contact, and her being confined to her room made us fear for her life.

After sending the email, my mom drove an hour north to the facility and tried to visit Memom to give her Christmas presents from the family. Of course, no one was allowed in the facility, so Mom had to leave the presents on a chair located in the vestibule. The aide we hired retrieved the gifts and took them to Memom's room, as she was not allowed to leave it. Mom stood outside the window, bundled in her hat and coat and winter gear since it was a chilly, gloomy day. Mom called the aide's personal cell phone rather than shouting through the window. Memom had a hard time hearing on speakerphone, so the aide repeated everything Mom said. As Mom pressed her face against the dirty window, she watched Memom open the presents. As an early Christmas present for me that year, my mom scheduled a makeover and photo session with my best friend from high school. We went to Trap Pond State Park with my Goldendoodle, Carter, to take pictures. I framed several for Memom to display in her apartment. In some respects, I am glad I was not there at the window to see her open them because Mom told me she could see a few tears fall from Memom's eyes as she saw the photos. On the other hand, I regret not being there for Memom to share some light in her darkest times. At that point, I didn't have much hope of seeing Memom for Christmas.

My mom's brother was power of attorney for Memom, and my mom was the medical power of attorney. Mom's sister was involved in the conversations about the holidays as well but did not have an official legal role. Her brother lives in Florida, where visitation was open for family members and, according to AARP, had the lowest COVID infection rates for staff and residents of facilities at that time. Even though it would mean I would have to travel far to see Memom,

I wanted her to have a normal, happy life with the ability to see family and friends. I was at my parents' house the weekend before Christmas, and I remember overhearing a conversation between my mom and her siblings. They were discussing buying a house in my uncle's neighborhood where my aunt from Colorado would move in with Memom. I knew as soon as I heard the conversation that this was just a pie-in-the-sky dream, and nothing would come of it. There was a fear that if we had Memom at our house for the holidays, we would expose her to COVID. I didn't understand the rationale behind the thought that her risk of getting sick would be higher in a house where fewer people came in and out than in the facility she lived in.

On Christmas Day 2020, we planned to use ViewClix to call Memom after our early dinner to watch her open her gifts. One of my biggest regrets, other than having her in the facility alone on Christmas Day, is not calling first thing in the day to say Merry Christmas. My aunt called early in the evening, and Memom was still sitting alone in a gray t-shirt with her hair unbrushed and no makeup on. With no visitation allowed, Memom couldn't spend time with anyone she loved for the first time in her 96 years of life. Viewing the screenshot of the video chat, I can remember thinking of Memom as old for the first time in my life. She looked crushed, spending the day isolated from friends and family. She had lost the option of getting dressed up for Christmas for the first time, too. Almost unrecognizable, I didn't even know Memom owned a gray t-shirt, as she usually wore nice nightgowns to bed. We called Memom at 7 p.m. and could not get her on the line. She was notorious her whole life for being a night owl—and that night, she chose to go to bed early.

After the holidays were over, my anxiety grew about not being able to see Memom. We knew she had a foot wound at this point, but no one in the family had been able to see the wound nor attend the doctor appointments. We hadn't been within a few feet of her since December 1st. I couldn't shake the feeling that something bad was going to happen. I called my uncle on January 19th to beg him to consider transferring Memom to an assisted living facility in Florida. Even though I wouldn't be able to see Memom, I hated knowing she was confined in a room devoid of social and family interaction. Memom had chosen to go to an assisted living facility on her own terms because she wanted to live as independently as possible while having some assistance and lots of social activities. Every costume event or party—count on Memom attending and being the star of the show. I had researched AARP on state COVID performance in both their death rate and their visitation policies. Since lots of elderly people retire to Florida, there was a plethora of options for facilities within a few miles of my uncle's home. At the time, I thought that since he was the power of attorney, he had the ultimate decision and decided to present a fact-based, reasonable position.

When I discussed it with my uncle in Florida, he disagreed due to his perception of how that state was handling the COVID-19 crisis. Some news networks and sources crucified Florida for their management of COVID-19 in not having strict lockdowns. Articles such as "America Didn't Give Up on COVID-19. Republicans Did" by Paul Krugman, published on June 25, 2020, in the *New York Times*, or "Even by Florida standards, Gov. Ron DeSantis is a COVID-19 catastrophe" by Lizette Alvarez on December 21, 2020, in *The Washington Post*, presented high-level information and division, including the nickname "DeathSantis" for the Governor. Unfortunately, by doing so, they did not share the data behind the results—just the perception that lockdowns were the only way to manage COVID. The phone conversation ended, and I emailed the research I put together to justify the proposed move on January 19, 2021.

Email written January 19, 2021:

I thought I'd pass along research and data on how each state is performing, specifically with the elderly in nursing homes and vaccination rates. I highly encourage everyone to read the investigation done by AARP on the impact of neglect and isolation of the elderly as well.

Florida has the lowest resident COVID-19 deaths- rate per 100 residents at 0.44. Delaware is at 1.02 and U.S. average is at 1.9. (source: https://www.aarp.org/ppi/issues/caregiving/info-2020/ nursing-home-covid-dashboard.html)

Vaccination rate:

Florida ranks 25th in the country at vaccination rate. Delaware is 42 (source: https://www.beckershospitalreview.com/public-health/ states-ranked-by-percentage-of-covid-19-vaccines-administered. html)

On January 22nd, I called Memom's lawyer's office to discuss a consultation about a potential lawsuit. I was prepared to sue the state of Delaware for violating nursing home resident rights. My mom told my uncle about the meeting, and he texted me that he would like to be a part of it. He said that despite our different ways of seeing how to take care of Memom, "we both want what is best for her." I shared that I was prepared to pay the $250 for an uninterrupted meeting with Memom's lawyer and said my uncle was not invited to the meeting. He said he understood, but the disagreement caused me to lose my relationship with my uncle, as we have not spoken since.

During the meeting with Memom's lawyer on January 25th, I referenced several examples of lack of care that I felt led to her wound issues:

- Confinement in her room each time there was a positive COVID case, with only approximately 20 feet of walking space from her bed to her recliner.
- Restriction from walks to the dining room or walks outside to get fresh air.
- Delivery of meals three times a day to Memom's recliner.

Severely restricted movement throughout the day led to a lack of blood flow to her extremities. This resulted in a lack of healing since healing any injury requires good blood flow.

I believed the residents' rights of long-term care facilities and services were violated during the pandemic (https://delcode.delaware.gov/title16/c011/sc02/index.html).

(1) Each resident shall have the right to receive considerate, respectful, and appropriate care, treatment, and services, in compliance with relevant federal and state law and regulations, recognizing each person's basic personal and property rights, which include dignity and individuality.

(14) a. Each resident may associate and communicate, including visits and visitation, privately and without restriction with persons and groups of the resident's own choice, on the resident's own or their initiative, at any reasonable hour.

(30) Each resident shall be free from verbal, physical, or mental abuse, cruel and unusual punishment, involuntary seclusion, withholding of monetary allowance, withholding of food, and deprivation of sleep.

(31) Each resident shall be free to make choices regarding activities, schedules, health care, and other aspects of the resident's life that are significant to the resident, as long as such choices are consistent with the resident's interests, assessments, and plan of care and do not

compromise the health or safety of the individual or other residents within the facility.

(32) Each resident has the right to participate in an ongoing program of activities designed to meet, in accordance with the resident's individualized assessments and plan of care, the resident's interests and physical, mental, and psychosocial well-being.

My mother joined the call with the lawyer and said she, too, believed the lack of movement contributed to Memom not being able to heal. Before the pandemic, my mom was able to attend Memom's cardiology appointments. Her cardiologist's mother had been in Memom's facility, so he was familiar with the layout of the facility. He told Memom that walking to the dining room from her room at least three times a day would be enough exercise to keep her healthy. Mom and I thought that if the cardiologist would write an order for three daily walks from her room to the dining room and if that plan was carefully implemented, Memom would heal faster and remain healthy. When I mentioned suing the state of Delaware, her lawyer said that the process would take so long that Memom would be dead before it helped her get the right to walk in the hallway. After the meeting, Mom and I decided that we would work with Memom's cardiologist to obtain a letter requesting accommodations for Memom. We never finalized the letter, however, due to Memom's hospitalization 10 days later.

I had the idea to sue the state because of another lawsuit in the spring of 2020. Patrick J. Murray of Delaware filed a lawsuit against Governor John Carney regarding his restrictions on access to beaches and the ban on short-term rentals and commercial lodging. According to *"Federal lawsuit targets Delaware coronavirus* restrictions," an article by Randall Chase published in AP News on May 15, 2020, the plaintiff "swore in an affidavit that he will suffer irreparable injury if he is unable to rent the couple's Dewey Beach condominium starting

Memorial Day weekend, because the rental income from the summer pays the mortgage for the year." Claiming that citizens' constitutional rights would be violated by not being able to make money from condo rentals would certainly be no more serious than claiming that a citizen's rights would be violated as they were denied access to reasonable ambulatory exercise rather than being restricted to a single resident's room for weeks on end. My logic was flawed. As stated in the article, there is a "least-restrictive-means test" in reference to government regulations. In my opinion, individual civil liberties had been violated by the government regulations for isolation. Thinking I had a case, I called the plaintiff's attorney's office and left a voicemail stating my concerns. Patrick J. Murray's wife, Julianne Murray, happened to be the lawyer representing him. No one from the attorney's office returned my call. I found it hard to believe that the mental safety of the elderly was less of a priority than rental income. I called several other law offices in an attempt to get a similar lawsuit started for government overreach but failed to get anyone to talk to me. It became clear profits were a priority over people. Julianne declared candidacy as a contender for governor in the 2020 election but lost to the incumbent, Governor Carney.

Long-term care concerns

At this point, I was calling anyone in administration in the State of Delaware whom I thought would listen to my concerns about the vaccine and about how long-term care facilities were being managed. Isolation and keeping families away from their loved ones had led to dire consequences. If residents were being required to have two vaccines before visitation policies would be relaxed, I would make it my mission to reach out to everyone who could speed up the process. My mother also decided to write to four local legislators about her experience on January 25, 2021, two days after she got her first vaccine.

Mom's letter

COVID19 Vaccination Issues

Dear Sir,

I am reaching out to you regarding our state's vaccination distribution. Last Tuesday evening I received an email message from Governor Carney's office announcing a weekend vaccination event for citizens 65 and older. Registration was to commence the following morning at 8:30.

The registration system crashed the next morning, but my daughter was able to circumvent the original link and register me and her grandmother for the weekend event at DMV.

My mother-in-law and uncle, both in their late 80's, were driven by our cousin to their 10:00 appointment. They arrived an hour early and waited in the vehicle line for four hours before receiving their vaccinations. It was a daunting ordeal for both of them and now they are reticent to repeat this for their booster shots, which are necessary to increase their immunity.

My appointment was at 3:00, so when I heard about the delays, I left home early and took my place in line on the shoulder of northbound 113 at 1:45. I was 1.8 miles south of DMV at that point. I spent the next five hours in my car stopping and starting as we crept toward the vaccine distribution site. We started single file, then were directed around the social services center in two lanes, subsequently merging into one lane three additional times.

In the DMV parking lot, I was approached by a healthcare worker who gave me a form to be completed as I drove slowly toward my destination in the dark. She informed me that their record system had crashed and they were unable to access my identity or the preliminary forms that I had filled out ahead of time regarding health issues, allergies, and other information pertinent to receiving any vaccine.

At the end point, I was asked to add my telephone number so that someone could contact me at a later date regarding my booster shot necessary at 28 days.

This is an insane and inhumane way to treat our most vulnerable population.

Please advocate for DHHS and our governor to look for alternative solutions to this plan. The vast majority of our senior citizens do not work during the week, cannot sit behind the wheel for 4 – 9 hours, and have difficulty navigating the Internet (especially when the system crashes).

There are better state models for our state to reference, in particular, West Virginia. They have a population of 1.7 million, their terrain is much more challenging than Delaware's both in area and infrastructure, and yet they are distributing 100% of their vaccine, have vaccinated their elderly (in long term care facilities and in the community) and will begin to offer vaccines to citizens in their 50's this week.

WVA strategy highlights:

- *They use their National Guard with people at a command center to coordinate distribution to small sites throughout their state where elders go for appointments*

- *They do not follow the federal plan, using local partnerships with small pharmacies and local medical centers as distribution points*
- *They DO NOT use mass distribution events (like the ones last weekend)*
- *Their underlying concern is to ACCOMMODATE the older people*
- *They use health care providers to identify persons at highest risk*
- *Their phone line/internet registration offers realtime updates and scheduling*
- *They use 100% of their vaccine allocations*
- *They place the highest emphasis on 70 and above as they recognize that those individuals have a 220% - 630% higher death rate from contracting COVID 19*

Please advocate for your most vulnerable citizens. My greatest fear is that the many senior citizens who did endure the hours-long waits last weekend will not want to repeat that experience to get their Pfizer or Moderna booster shots in 21 or 28 days and that will lead to a 50% reduction in their protection from this deadly disease.

Time is of the essence.

Lucilla Esham

One of the local newspapers, the Delaware State News, ran an article on the front page regarding my mom's experience with the vaccination process. Media attention seemed to put pressure on the vaccine administrators to improve the process. However, only one of the legislators responded to her email, and it was over a month later.

Representative Hensley meeting January 2021

In addition to writing and calling people at the state offices, I was in contact with my local representative. I attended Kevin Hensley's town hall meeting in the Odessa Fire Hall on January 12, 2021. Due to lockdowns, it was the first meeting held in public in a while. The meeting started with discussions on the challenge of getting access to the vaccine. Approximately 30 residents of Middletown attended the meeting, sitting in chairs spaced out three feet apart. Most residents were retired and living in the local community. Representative Hensley spoke of the lack of vaccines nationwide and the priority population. At the end of January 2021, the target population for the first phase of vaccines would be residents 65 and older and front-line workers. I mentioned other states, such as Florida, that were able to get vaccines distributed faster than the state of Delaware and how my mom and I called someone every day trying to get Memom vaccinated. Hoping emotion would get attention, I discussed how, on Christmas Day, no one even came to make sure Memom was dressed and had her hearing aids in. My voice shook and tears started as I described this being the worst year of my life; I shared how Memom could not get to a doctor's appointment because everyone was on quarantine. I explained my family's fear that her vaccination priority would be lost if she was removed from her current setting. This fear impacted our decision to keep her in the facility. Each Delaware U.S. representative I reached out to simply blamed the federal government. I knew that two-thirds of the state's vaccine inventory was not being administered despite a 30-day shelf life. The state of Delaware government website had a Delaware Environmental Public Health Tracking Network with data on vaccines received from the federal government and how many had been distributed to Delaware residents. I monitored this website daily, hoping the state distribution would improve. Two days later, an article, "Health care workers report trouble getting vaccines in Delaware," by Holveck and Gamard in *The News Journal*, described state officials "struggling to make sure the state's front-line health care workers are vaccinated before moving on to more widespread vaccinations." This included delays for residents 65 and older. According to the article, less than half of Delaware's doses had been administered.

The meeting continued with discussions around how the legislative session would be conducted since Delaware was still in a state of emergency and with discussions on local items such as infrastructure. Representative Collins, from Sussex County, introduced House Bill 245, which requires the Legislature to approve extensions of the Governor's state of emergency order if an emergency lasts more than 180 days. At this point, the executive branch (Governor) was able to extend the emergency order and all mandates associated with it without input from the General Assembly or citizens. Mandates included banning families from visiting loved ones in long-term care facilities and acute care hospitals. I questioned Representative Hensley regarding his perspective; he was supportive of the bill yet did not sign on as a co-sponsor. Over three years later, in April 2024, this bill was discussed in the House Administration Committee Meeting but did not receive enough signatures to release it from committee.

Road issues, standing water, and Department of Transportation discussions dominated the remainder of the representative's topics in the town hall meeting until open comment. Toward the end of the meeting, a lady requested that an elder caucus be established as our state has other groups such as women and children represented. She mentioned neglect in long-term care facilities and the need to tackle the issue of neglect. I left the meeting shocked that conversations about grocery stores, Wawa (a convenience store), and roadwork were among the greatest worries of attendees. Two days later, Memom and other residents of the assisted living facility received their first COVID vaccine. Mom and I saw this as the first step toward more frequent visitation.

State of Delaware Calls Before Hospitalization

Desperate for visitation rights with Memom and for ways to stop the continued trauma of isolation for all residents, I called a new department each day. I begged for help and lobbied for their understanding regarding the need for changes. Sometimes a person would answer, and other times I left a voicemail, which meant there was about a fifty percent chance that someone would call me back. One state employee told me she didn't think residents would ever be able to safely return to the dining hall at full capacity and that the residents' routines would be permanently altered. I found it especially disturbing that dictating and influencing restrictions on our lives had given up hope that we would ever get back to normal. She shared that her daughter was a nurse and saw firsthand the devastating impact of isolation on elders. As a result of that conversation, I wrote an email titled "Lockdown Isolation" to the Department of Public Health on January 19, 2021:

Good afternoon,

I am writing on behalf of my grandmother who is in a long-term care facility in Dover. Can you tell me what the state guidelines are for when residents are allowed to leave their rooms? My grandmother received the first vaccine last Thursday and we were told then she would be able to go to the dining hall and eat outside of her room. Also that activities with other residents would resume. Now the director is saying the state of Delaware has said residents are not allowed to interact with each other indefinitely.

I am concerned about the impact of isolation and her spending hours alone. Please let me know the state guidelines on resident interaction after the vaccine. Feel free to call me.

Thank you,

Candace Esham

Finally, on Sunday, January 24, 2021, I received a call from the Executive Director of the Delaware Nursing Home Resident Quality Assurance Commission (DNHRQAC). I almost couldn't believe a state employee was calling me on a Sunday since I had been hitting dead ends. We focused on the issues of visitation, my fear of the impact isolating Memom from family and friends had on her mental state, and several questions around vaccines. As I did during my representative's Town Hall, I shared the success story of the West Virginia vaccination rollout for the elderly living in long-term care facilities, despite the state's challenges of being primarily rural and having smaller pharmacies. She was knowledgeable about contacts for the state health department's plan for long-term care facilities and the vaccination program, and she committed to following up on questions I emailed her as a summary from the call.

1. *What are facilities doing to ensure third party vendors have access to the vaccine?*
2. *What is the follow up plan for individuals who were vaccinated in Georgetown yesterday after the system crashed? My mother received the vaccine but received a cancellation email last night. She wrote her name and number on a paper at the DMV. How will she schedule her second dose?*
3. *What will be done differently for the second vaccine administration to avoid 5 hour waits in the car?*

4. *What is the post vaccine re-open plan for LTCF? Will dining and activities? Here is an article on how West Virginia is so successful in their vaccination rate: ["Why West Virginia's Winning The Race to Get COVID-19 Vaccine Into Arms" by Yuki Noguchi, January 7, 2021 in NPR] https://www.npr.org/sections/health-shots/2021/01/07/954409347/why-west-virginias-winning-the-race-to-get-covid-19-vaccine-into-arms*

I appreciate all the time you took to listen to my concerns. Please let me know if I can do anything to help.

Thanks,

Candace Esham

Email received 1/26/21

Hi Candace - As a follow-up to your questions, please note responses that appear in red:

1. *What are facilities doing to ensure 3rd party vendors have access to the vaccine?*

Response: The facilities could have included them in the vaccinations with the federal pharmacy program. Many of these individuals have been included in the various clinics as part of 1A.

2. *What is the follow up plan for individuals who were vaccinated in Georgetown yesterday after the system crashed? My mother received the vaccine but received a cancellation email last night. She wrote her name and number on a paper at the DMV. How will she schedule her second dose?*

Response: The system did not crash. The laptops were not working properly because of the extreme cold temperatures so they decided to use paper forms. We are aware that some people received a message in error that their appointments were cancelled and we ask them to disregard that notice. We have her information on the forms and it will be entered into our electronic system. At this time, we are not scheduling second doses in advance due to limited supply of the vaccine. Also, she does not have to get her second does at the same location, only needs to have the same type of vaccine (Moderna). By the time she is eligible for her second dose in 28 – 42 days, she will have more options for places to go including several pharmacies, others holding drive thru events and possibly primary care providers in addition to state run drive thru events like Saturdays.

3. *What will be done differently for the second vaccine to avoid 5 hour waits in the car?*

Response: The Department of Public Health learned a lot from Saturday's event. We started vaccinating before appointment times began so we were never behind, we sent out instructions Sunday morning to people with appointments to ask them to make sure they had filled out the pre-screening questionnaire online which was causing delays onsite when staff had to complete that for people, we added additional state police resources for traffic control. For most of the day Sunday, the wait was under half an hour, and we anticipate the lessons learned will carry forward to future events.

4. *What is the post vaccine re-open plan for LTCF? When will residents be resuming dining and activities?*

Response: The post vaccination plan is currently under review as it is still too early to determine the effectiveness of the vaccine. At this time, facilities that have not had a COVID 19 outbreak for at least 14 days are eligible for dining and activities with precautions in place.

Please let me know if you have any additional questions. I'd be happy to ask :).

I'd also like to know if you've heard back from Ombudsman?

Information about the Delaware Nursing Home Residents Quality Assurance Commission: https://courts.delaware.gov/dnhrqac/.

Have a great evening,
Margaret Bailey
State of Delaware
DNHRQAC
Executive Director

Media before hospitalization

Media attention drives policy changes, and I sought media attention because I believed the isolation of long-term care residents needed to stop. Front page news stories influence conversations in the community, which usually cause engaged constituents to call or write their local legislators. If an issue isn't well known or broadly supported, there is no urgency for change.

The State of Delaware has two major newspapers, The News Journal and the Delaware State News. I reached out to a reporter from each newspaper, hoping one of them would see the importance of covering the issues. Two News Journal reporters, Brandon Holveck and Sarah Gamard, wrote "Health care workers report trouble getting vaccines in Delaware" on January 14, 2021. It described the struggles of ensuring front-line health care workers received the vaccine before residents over 65 and some essential workers. The vaccine phases were as follows:

- *Phase 1A: Health care personnel, emergency medical service agencies, and long-term care residents and staff.*
- *Phase 1B: People 65 and older, and front-line essential workers such as firefighters, police officers, teachers, U.S. Postal Service workers, grocery store workers, correctional officers, public transit employees, childcare providers, and food processing workers.*
- *Phase 1C: People 16-64 with high-risk medical conditions, people in high-risk group settings such as shelters or group homes, and other essential workers such as transportation and logistics employees, food service workers, construction workers, finance, IT and communications employees, members of the media, legal workers, and public safety workers.*
- *Phase 2: People 50-64, people 16-49 with moderate-risk medical conditions, and essential workers not included in Phase 1.*
- *Phase 3: People 16-49 and essential workers not included in Phase 2.*
- *Phase 4: Anyone who didn't have access to vaccines in prior phases.*

Complaints of having to know someone to be able to get the vaccine were prevalent throughout the state. As of Tuesday, January 12, 2021, 42 of the state's 188 long-term care facilities had started vaccinating residents according to the phases outlined in the article. Unlike West Virginia's vaccination program for long-term care, which successfully utilized small local pharmacies, Delaware officials decided to use a federal-level pharmacy.

In an email, I reached out to the co-author of the article, Brandon Holveck, on January 22, 2021.

Good afternoon Brandon,

I read your article on the covid vaccine plan. I had two ideas for stories that I think residents would be interested in.

What is the plan for long term care facilities post COVID vaccine? My grandmother is in one in Dover and has been confined to her room for months. The isolation and lack of ability to walk even to the dining hall has caused a major decline in her physical and emotional health. Christmas day she sat alone, undressed (pajamas), hair unbrushed, and no hearing aids in. We have a video box in her room so that's how I know. I was told by the state board of health that the isolation plan is "indefinite" because the vaccine is not 100% effective. On October, 22, 2020, the governor of Florida lifted the restrictions on visitors with specific criteria since Florida residents recognized the impact of isolation (source https://floridahealthcovid19.gov/nursing-homes/) Florida has the lowest resident COVID-19 deaths with a rate per 100 residents of 0.44. Delaware is at 1.02. source: https://www.aarp.org/ppi/issues/caregiving/info-2020/nursing-home-covid-dashboard.html

Why is the vaccination rate of Delaware so slow? Delaware is 28th in the nation in vaccination rate with only 46.31% of doses received administered (source: https://www.beckershospitalreview.com/public-health/

states-ranked-by-percentage-of-covid-19-vaccines-administered.
html) Why aren't we moving forward with a distribution plan
like West Virginia (source: https://www.npr.org/sections/health-
shots/2021/01/07/954409347/why-west-virginias-winning-the-
race-to-get-covid-19-vaccine-into-arms).

I am concerned with the path forward in this state and am reach-
ing out to local representatives as well as the board of health.
Most people are shocked when I provide the data and I think your
readers would be interested in it. I would be happy to discuss or
provide more info via email or phone.

Thanks,

Candace Esham

I sent a similar email on January 22, 2021, to a journalist with the *Delaware State News* after reading his article on the vaccine plan. Surprisingly, the next day I heard back from him and was hopeful a story would be published. Initially, he believed a story about the impact of isolation would be worthwhile, and we exchanged several emails about that. The article about the lengthy vaccination process my mother experienced made the front cover of the *Delaware State News* a few days after I contacted the journalist, but the story about long-term care facilities was not moving forward quickly.

Emails with Kyla- Life Enrichment Coordinator
at the assisted living facility

We had limited information about how Memom was handling the imposed isolation or her health. When my mom called the nurse to ask about Memom, often the answers were short and terse. The life enrichment coordinator cared deeply about Memom and would send us updates in emails. Even though these emails didn't describe what was actually going on in the facility, this was our only source of information. She would visit with Memom and attempt to assist her in leaving her room when it was allowed.

August 28, 2020

Hi Kyla!

What a crazy week. I am so thankful I got to spend time with Memom on Wednesday despite the circumstances. The entire staff at Christiana who were taking care of her that I met were amazing. She is so strong and I'm so thankful her internal bleeding stopped. I was able to sit with her in the ED and get her checked into the ICU. She was telling everyone about her helicopter ride. I miss her so much. I am hoping to come do porch visits once its cooler. I blacked out and had a seizure a couple of weeks ago due to the heat I think so I haven't been outside during the day much. I am still working from home so that is nice.

Please send a picture of your new furry family member! Very excited for you guys! Carter is loving me being home.

I told Memom we have so much to look forward to when we can have events again. You always plan the best activities. I know they will be modified for awhile but you always make things fun!

Here is one of my favorite pictures of the three of us. If you need anything else let me know! I took Memom's purse and clothes to my house and Carter could smell Memom. He definitely misses visiting too. He gets spoiled with all the love there. Ann keeps little pieces of bacon in her walker for him! Haha.

Thank you for being creative with the grandparent's day celebration. Hope to see you sometime!

Candace

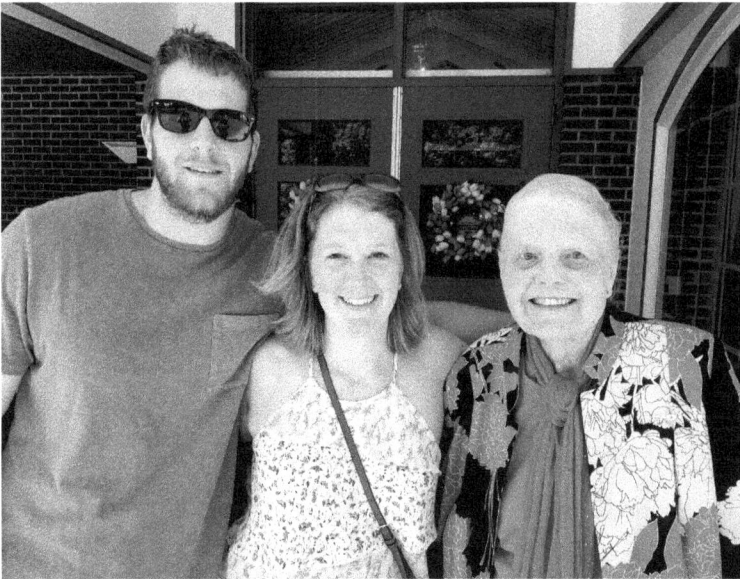

January 24, 2021

Hi Kyla!

Mom sent me the pictures of you walking with Memom yesterday. The hot chocolate sounded amazing! Definitely was the perfect day for that. I wanted to thank you for always thinking of the details to make the day special for Memom and the residents

there. I truly believe you and Sheri are Memom's angels. I am
continuing to pray for everyone's health and to get back to the fun
days. I have so many wonderful memories with the events you've
organized and with Memom and the other residents there. They
are all so special and I know you do a lot for everyone. Carter and
I miss everyone dearly. When I say Memom is here on the video
when we talk, Carter runs to the door thinking she is coming to our
house. I forget if I told you but when I picked up her clothes and her
purse from the hospital in August when she fell, he managed to get
her bow out of the bag and was carrying it around. He knew it was
Memom's things. He didn't mess it up just gently took it around the
house. He has such a tender heart. Hope you and your family are
well. Wishing for the brighter days ahead.

Candace

Hospitalization

February 4, 2021, was supposed to be a day of celebration. Memom received her second COVID vaccine, and this meant we would be able to see her more often according to the facility's visitation policy. We would be able to take her out for a meal and spend more quality time with her. On the morning of February 4th, my mom got a call from the nurse at the facility. The nurse stated that Memom needed to go to the hospital immediately due to redness starting from her infected toe, which was spreading up her leg. In celebration of the second vaccine for residents, the facility decided to have a Mardi Gras party. Memom dressed in a deep purple suit, which was one of her favorite colors to wear. She was ready to go down the hall to the Bistro and enjoy music, food, and fun. When the nurse approached her about going to the hospital, she didn't understand why she had to go. Nothing could stop Memom from want-ing to go to a party and have a good time. They decided to send her via ambulance after lunch and her second vaccine shot.

At this point, we had still not seen the wound or had any indication of how serious the situation was. Mom and I thought that if the wound was serious enough for hospital care, we would have had more frequent communication about it. February is prime flu season, so we worried about Memom catching a respiratory illness in the waiting room. This was her first hospital visit where we couldn't be with her upon admis-sion. Nurses and doctors updated the electronic chart with limited information, but I monitored all updates to learn what was happening. The admission notes included a photo of Memom's foot wound, which showed deep purple discoloration of her second toe and a deep black scab on her large toe. Although I am not medically trained, the picture made me wonder how anyone could let a wound progress to this point without prior acute hospital care. Angered by the lack of urgency to get Memom help, I immediately reached out to the State of Delaware and my local representative to file a complaint. At the time, I believed Memom would recover from the wound and go back to the assisted living facility. My main concern still was ensuring families could visit residents in long-term care facilities to prevent resident isolation

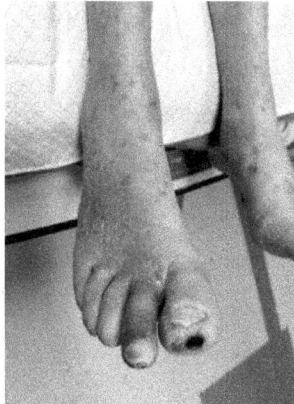

trauma and ensure quality care was provided.

We tried to set up a FaceTime call on Saturday, February 6th, but the three times we called during the 12-hour day shift, the nurse said she hadn't gotten a chance to charge the iPad. I still don't understand what was so hard about making it possible for us to communicate with Memom. Human compassion seemed to be lacking in the nurses we interacted with. It seemed that they didn't want the extra burden of families being involved in their loved one's care. At this point, I had not seen how "busy" the nurses were and tried to give them the benefit of the doubt. Later, during Memom's hospital stay, I saw nurses with time to play on their phones, apparently not busy with patient care. This made it even harder to believe that charging an iPad presented an unreasonable challenge. We only placed one family call per shift to try to streamline communications, but even that seemed too cumbersome for staff.

Due to her sepsis diagnosis, Memom started antibiotics. The podiatrist was concerned about how much damage the infection had done to her foot and scheduled Memom for an MRI for a vascular study on February 6, 2021, to determine if amputation was feasible. She moved in the MRI, invalidating the test results. It was unclear whether the podiatrist discussed vascular health with Dr. Shuck, her cardiologist, to determine amputation feasibility. With the confusion Memom had due to sepsis, even if we had the opportunity to talk with her, we wouldn't have gotten the full picture of the options and risks. We relied on once-a-shift updates from the nurses and had no idea how life-threatening the wound was. At this time, we thought the worst-case situation was a minor amputation. On Sunday, February 7th, my parents were at my house; we were hoping one of us would be able to visit Memom. My mom's brother, who lived in Florida, was considering flying up to visit Memom in the hospital. For some reason, the staff was in initial agreement that the family member flying in from Florida would be the one eligible to visit. I overheard a call between my mom and her two siblings; they were discussing the impact amputation would have on Memom's ability to walk. Given the information we had at the time, her siblings were not in agreement with amputation.

Finally, on Monday, February 8th, my mom, dad, and I were able to FaceTime together with Memom. My parents were at my house so we could all talk together since the rules mandated a limit of one FaceTime call per day. Memom was awake and reading the newspaper. She was looking out the window of her room and said she wished it was a view of the beach. The podiatrist came in during the FaceTime call; we reviewed the plan of care and wound status. He said the antibiotics were working and surgery would be difficult as her wound may not heal, so Mom and I assumed that meant everything was going to be okay. Given his explanation of the risks, we thought the least risky option for her health was to proceed with strong antibiotics. My mom gave the other FaceTime spots on the next few days to her brother and sister, so I did not see how quickly Memom declined in just a few short days. Each shift, I would log online to access Memom's patient records from the hospital to try to interpret her status. Luckily, I had friends in healthcare, and I could ask what certain phrases meant. I could also develop questions for doctors or nurses whenever we got an opportunity to speak with them. Relying solely on provider notes in a portal didn't give us any indication that she only had days to live.

On Tuesday, February 9th, I still believed Memom would recover from her wound, and my biggest fear was sending her back to the assisted living facility without being able to ensure her safety. Restrictions on visitation and family involvement did not seem to be improving at all, so I felt the need to try to get policies changed. Despite being exhausted from worrying about Memom, I attended my local representative's

Town Hall meeting the morning of the 9th.Community members once again sat spaced out in the Odessa Fire Hall. Representative Hensley began the meeting with discussions on the vaccine and concerns with distribution. Sitting in the front row with a notebook, I raised my hand and brought up West Virginia's plan "Save Our Wisdom," which effectively rolled out the vaccine to residents of all 214 long-term care facilities by the end of December 2020. Meanwhile, not all facilities in Delaware had received doses in December. Despite locking out families and keeping residents isolated most of the time, 39 of the 85 residents and 23 staff members in Memom's assisted living facility had tested positive for COVID. While Memom never tested positive, each outbreak increased her risk of infection, restricted her to her room, and left the facility short-staffed.

I brought an 8x11 picture of Memom's foot to show the representative and meeting attendees. Ensuring the people in the room knew the wound was a direct result of isolation, lack of care, and locking out loved ones was a critical point I hoped to make. My notes included the cost we were paying—an extra $2,000 a month for an aide, information on Florida lifting the restriction in October of 2020, and safety statistics from AARP. Angered by the lack of knowledge from decision-makers, I questioned why best practices from other states were not known. I referenced benchmarking car safety standards before purchasing a vehicle, but key players in COVID policymaking were not doing so amidst a pandemic. I contrasted consumer reliance on available benchmarks for car safety standards with the lack of availability of benchmarks in formulating COVID policies. Raising a hard copy of the latest AARP pamphlet with the front-page article titled "An American Tragedy," I emphasized the national crisis of neglect in long-term care facilities. The article, published December 3, 2020, described the lobbying effort to protect facilities against lawsuits as the main priority, despite the ongoing harm to residents. Representative Hensley stated he would keep working on behalf of residents of facilities.

Another meeting attendee stated ombudsmen were not allowed in facilities, eliminating a key avenue through which residents might have their concerns addressed. She also described bedsores her disabled, non-verbal granddaughter developed in a hospital setting due to a lack of turning her in bed. Hospital restrictions prevented the family from checking on their loved one; neglect occurred in acute care settings as well. State budget discussions continued for the next 30 minutes; no discussions for programs to support the elderly made the highlights. The status of the new Wawa, a convenience store in the Northeast of the U.S., was "top of mind," according to the representative. My mind could only focus on worrying about Memom; I couldn't wait for the day when I cared about a new gas station. I drove back to my house after the meeting to begin my workday.

The hospital policy at the time was only one FaceTime call per day per patient, so I didn't have the chance to speak with Memom or see how quickly her mental capabilities were declining due to sepsis and pain. My assumption was that the antibiotics were working like they had been when she was in the hospital in 2019. I believed the hospitalist or podiatrist would call us with concerns. When I read that her toe fell off in bed on Wednesday, February 10th, I knew we needed to change the plan. It never occurred to me to ask how her pain was being managed before her toe fell off, as I trusted healthcare providers would make the best decision for Memom. I started questioning and doubting that her foot would heal with just antibiotics at this point. Gangrene and amputation were even noted by Hippocrates, who lived somewhere between 450 and 380 BCE. How a patient's toe fell off in a hospital setting really disturbed me. It caused me to challenge Memom's plan of care. I believed her medical team did not give her a chance and saw her as expendable. In my opinion, they made a financial decision since the podiatrist does not get paid if something happens in the operating room.

By the end of the day on Friday, February 12th, Mom had asked Dr. Schuck, the cardiologist, if Memom could handle the amputation; he said yes. My mom had to facilitate the discussions between the providers; there was agreement between her cardiologist and podiatrist that a partial amputation of her toe would take place on Monday, February 15th.

On Saturday, February 13th, my mother received a call from the Progressive Care Unit (PCU) nurse responsible for Memom's care; she asked that we get to the hospital to see how much pain Memom was in. We had asked to visit earlier in the week; that request was denied. This was one of the worst days of my life. When we got to the room, Memom was thrashing in pain and had lost the ability to speak words. Her eyes were rolling around in her head, and she was screaming in pain. I have nightmares reliving seeing her in that pain; I have never observed such a lack of care in my life. The nurse stood there and asked my mother and me when Memom's advanced directive was done; she asked whether she should be full code or DNR (do not resuscitate). We explained that my grandmother made this decision to be full code herself four years ago after she was admitted to Kent General for a UTI and given a DNR band. Since Memom was a geriatric nurse, she knew the purpose of an advanced directive and made sure hers reflected her wishes. She was only on Tylenol and antibiotics at this point. Her second toe had fallen off in her hospital bed on Wednesday, February 10th. We did not stay long, as it was hard to watch her thrashing in pain. We changed her to DNR after that visit and demanded pain medication. She was transferred to the Intensive Care Unit (ICU) that evening.

On Sunday, February 14th, the hospital called us again and said Memom would pass away within a few hours. We were allowed up to four visitors, so Dad, Mom, and I went to spend some time with her, thinking this would be our goodbye. Visiting hours were limited to immediate family members of patients for whom they thought death was imminent. We arrived at the hospital and checked in at the front desk, where they required us to take our temperature, and they issued new masks. Since Memom had MRSA, we donned gloves and a plastic gown over our regular clothes. I left my purse and belongings in the car, since MRSA is very contagious and can live on surfaces for months. A piece of paper served as our pass to the ICU. Normal visiting hours were 4 to 8 p.m., but since the nurses thought Memom might pass away before then, we arrived around 11 a.m.

When I walked through the double doors of the ICU area, I noticed the command center desk, where a nurse watched a TV show on her phone. Because I was so quiet walking through the door, she didn't notice me, then hid that she was watching a show on her phone. Even though I should've been focused on thinking about Memom and how I wanted to spend time with her, all I could think about was the façade of busyness. In reality, over our four days in the hospital, nurses often sat looking at their phones.

Once Memom was transferred to the ICU, they stopped all fluids and started morphine. After donning the gown and gloves, we slid back the door to Memom's room and went inside. She was not speaking or awake while we were there, but she'd squeeze my hand when I was talking with her. I talked to her like I knew she could hear me. I didn't want any negative talk and made sure she knew we were doing everything we could for her. When we walked in, her vitals weren't great, but, once she heard our voices, her heart rate and blood pressure became normal. The day before, she had been in so much pain and thrashing that I don't even remember holding her hand. First, I sat down next to her, held her hand, and told her I loved her. Feeling her squeeze my hand was helpful; I knew she could hear me and knew I was there. We asked her nurse to put her on more regular pain medication since she still seemed uncomfortable. I don't remember the entirety of the conversations, but, at one point, I needed a break and walked downstairs to the lobby area. Once I disposed of the gown and gloves, I took the elevator downstairs and found an area with chairs by the window. No one was sitting there, and no one walked by the area since we were there outside of normal visiting hours. My parents stayed with Memom. After about 30 minutes of trying to clear my head, I went back upstairs. We spent a few hours watching her and left.

Even though we were drained from thinking it was goodbye, we kept our dinner reservations at a local golf course. We decided Memom wouldn't have wanted us to cancel our plans and focused on hoping she would make it through. Even though the nurses let us see Memom because they thought the end of her life was near, I still had faith she might recover if the antibiotics kept working. Since her vital signs returned to normal when she knew we were in the room, I had hope. Memom was a fighter and never wanted anyone to worry about her. No matter what she was going through, she would always say, "I'm fine; go enjoy your day!" It didn't matter whether she was in the emergency room a few times before or if she was having a regular day with Bingo and time with friends. The only thing she cared about was for me to have a good day. She gave me a plaque that hangs in my bathroom; it says, "Do one thing every day that makes you happy." That was truly her wish for everyone. During dinner, we focused on her love of life and her strength.

The next morning, we woke up to no updates on her chart. Initially, when I spoke with the nurse responsible for Memom's care that day, he told me about her heart monitor; her vitals were fine. I questioned him as to whether he had the right patient since I knew ICU nurses were responsible for two patients. He was adamant that I didn't know what I was talking about until I asked him to check her birthday on file. Then he realized he was in the wrong room, updating me on the wrong patient. Luckily, I had worked in a hospital before and had several friends who worked in healthcare, so I knew enough to question him. We asked if Mom and I could come visit during the day due to the weather since we had the day before; we were told yes.

I was staying at my parents' house, so I drove my mom to the hospital an hour away. We assumed the two of us could visit since we had the day before. When we got there, the front desk staff told us we were there outside of visiting hours. The desk manager called the nurse manager, who said I was not approved to visit. I asked to speak with her. She said I should feel lucky I got to see my grandmother the day before since a few weeks ago no visitors were allowed. I asked why I could see her yesterday but not today; she responded that my grand-mother was "not actively dying today," so only my mother could visit. Medical providers use terminology like "actively dying" to describe patient status among colleagues, but it should never be used in that way to family members. Before this conversation, I was only focused on getting Memom out of the hospital, not discussing the events leading to the wound, but I'd had enough of suppressing my anger. In the lobby of the hospital, over the phone, I explained in detail how unlucky I felt about the trauma the assisted living facility put Memom and my family through. Tired of the excuses and of the healthcare workers I had interacted with making me feel guilty over my level of caring for Memom, I described each incident that resulted in more suffering for her. Even though most people would have apologized for speaking to a family member this way, the nurse manager simply gave in and let one of us up to see Memom. I was told to wait in the car since I couldn't sit in the vestibule area because the front desk clerk declared "people walk around all the time with COVID." I waited in the parking garage while my mother visited because according to the front desk attendant, I "could get COVID" from sitting in the chair I sat in the day before.

On Tuesday morning the 16th, Memom had still not received any fluids in her IV since Saturday the 13th. On Tuesday, Memom was assigned a new nurse. Out of all the medical providers I encountered during her stay, his is the only name I remember. Tyler hung a bag of fluids for Memom and discussed with the doctor the need for fluids on a regular basis. He said hospital policy would allow him to hang a 20 ml bag of fluid without consulting a doctor first.

Mom and I drove up during the 4 to 8 pm visiting hours, and once again they only let one person in. Mom wanted me to go in so I could talk with the nurse in person and see what was going on, since on Sunday we had been told Memom had hours to live. We still hoped that her body was fighting the infection and that she could have the amputation performed.

When I got up to the ICU, Tyler wanted to know about Memom's life, so I showed him pictures and told him about how passionate she was about nursing. I know Memom would have liked him. Even though I was given a visiting pass from the front desk security with specific times on it, Tyler told me to stay as long as I wished. Mom waited in the car since we were told only one person could come in. I didn't know it would be her last day before walking into the room, but I was the last family member to be with Memom. I've heard of family members waiting until everyone they loved could see them before they passed away. This was a Tuesday night, and she had not been conscious since Saturday. She looked emaciated, with cheeks sunken and ridges in her skull visible. The difference from Sunday to Tuesday was shocking. I knew she could hear me and feel my presence. During that last visit, I held her hand, but she was no longer able to squeeze mine. Each breath she took was labored, and I didn't know if it would be her last. I told

74

her if she wanted to fight to live, we would give her the best chance possible—but if she wanted to let go, I would understand. Sitting with her for over an hour, I talked about how much having her not only as a grandmother but as a role model meant to me. As each minute passed, I could tell she was barely holding on to life. I could tell Memom was ready to go, and it felt like she was holding on to see her son and other daughter. The day before, Mom had walked in on the minister using FaceTime with my mom's brother and sister and overheard them discussing the funeral. We knew they would not come to see Memom alive for fear of catching COVID on a plane. The hardest conversation I had during that time was one where I was the only one speaking. I held Memom's hand and told her that so many people loved her throughout the years. I told her I knew she was tired and that I would be okay without her, even though I would miss her. Praying she wouldn't stop breathing in front of me, I also told her no one else was coming, so she didn't have to hold on anymore if she was ready to go. I gave her a hug and told her I would see her later, knowing this would be the last time I would see her on Earth.

As I was walking to the elevator, I saw two people leaving another patient's room; they were looking for the lobby. Their son was waiting there, in the same lobby I was told I couldn't sit in. It never made sense to me how another family was allowed more visitors than ours that day. I felt horrible that my mom wasn't able to be the last one to say goodbye, but we were just taking it day by day. I am thankful one of my friends is a hospice nurse and helped walk me through the hospital charts each day so I could ask good questions to make sure Memom was comfortable. Seeing how much Memom had declined since Sunday was horrible. It was awful to be there by myself. I am grateful I was able to talk with her, but it was the hardest thing I have ever had to do. She didn't even look like herself with her sunken cheeks and ashy gray skin. I told her no one else was coming to see her and that if she was ready to let go, then I would let her go. I heard my dad's phone ring at about 11:30 pm and I knew she had passed.

Based on records we obtained after her death, Memom had an even more traumatic hospital stay than we could have imagined. I waited to review these records until January 2024 because I was not ready to relive the events or find out more about the hospital stay. People say timing is everything, and I believe the timing was right for me to give feedback and for the hospital to receive it. Despite the horrific events in the hospital, I do believe that the administration now has programs in place to prevent these same issues from happening to other patients and families. I am grateful I did not let these events go without addressing them.

The Dover EMS notes on February 4th at 1309 indicated that Memom had dementia as well as a "Do Not Resuscitate" (DNR) order. She injured her left and right arms on the 6th and 12th, respectively, from pulling her IV out. From the evening of Wednesday, February 10th, through the evening of Thursday, February 11th, Memom was physically restrained at the wrists and ankles due to hallucinations, agitation, and confusion. She was deemed to be a danger to herself and others. An occupational therapist worked with Memom on February 5th and not again until February 10th. The decline in her assessed abilities was extreme. On the morning of the 5th, she was able to stand and walk without assistance other than a walker. By the afternoon of the 10th, the notes state Memom "screamed and clutched onto the bed rails, scream-ing she does not want to fall." She screamed to be laid back in bed, and no further activities were performed. Notes in the pain assessment section mentioned advanced dementia the morning of February 11th, which had never been one of her diagnoses prior to the sepsis infection. She was never seen by a neurologist to diagnose this, just assumed by the nurse notes. Confusion and agitation are symptoms displayed by people with dementia, but they are also indicative of patients with severe infections.

Memom's pain assessment score changed to "critical-care pain" according to the assessment tool on February 12th. Prior to the "advanced dementia" pain assessment score, Memom assessed her pain consistently at zero out of ten. No pain medication, not even ibuprofen or acetaminophen, was administered to Memom during the entire hospital stay until morphine injections began when she was transferred to the ICU on the evening of February 13th.

We didn't receive the notes from the facility until March 11, 2021; her foot wound was hidden by the facility and the aide at that time. Memom is dead because we weren't aware of her medical health, even after my mom asked about Memom's care. I will never forget how she sat alone in her pajamas with her hair unbrushed and no hearing aids in on Christmas Day. My mother discussed removing Memom, but her brother and sister disagreed. Also, Memom had said she wanted to stay in the facility with the activities director and her aide. Fear of the unknown is crippling and paralyzing.

On September 11, 2020, she weighed 149 lbs.; on 12/8/20, she weighed 138 lbs. Anyone, no matter their age, kept in a room for weeks at a time, not given a choice to shower or get dressed, sitting in darkness with the blinds shut—anyone will suffer physically and mentally. Memom had hope for the vaccine and for the good times ahead. She carried my brother's wedding invitation in her purse (he was getting married June 12, 2021), and two new dresses hung in her closet, ready to be worn during the wedding festivities. Upset that she was missing a post-vaccine Mardi Gras party, she reluctantly agreed to go to the hospital. Through months of isolation from family, she remained hopeful. I expressed my concerns to state officials over the trauma residents have experienced due to required isolation. Any family who has a loved one in a facility needs access to the records. We will look back on the pandemic and realize how badly these decisions mandating isolation impacted the elderly.

After she was gone

Exhausted from seeing Memom suffer, I went to bed early on Tuesday, February 16th. I was still staying with my parents as I did not want to be alone and wanted to support them. My mom was the point of contact for the hospital, but her phone was on silent and she was sleeping. We heard my dad's cell phone ring downstairs around 11:30 pm. I knew it had to be bad news. My uncle called to tell us the hospital notified him Memom had passed away. Mom went downstairs to get the news, and she came to my room afterward. Even though I knew Memom couldn't hold on any longer, I began uncontrollably sobbing over losing her. I felt like she had suffered unnecessarily and had so much more life left to live. Thinking of Memom carrying my brother's wedding invitation in her purse and her two dresses hanging in her closet, I felt robbed of future memories with her. Memom had lived a healthy life. To think that people didn't get her the help she needed was inconceivable. I sat on my mom's bed, hugging her while I cried until my eyes were swollen.

Eventually, I went back to my bedroom and fell asleep for a couple of hours. I was still working remotely and had a meeting online the next morning. I remember coming down the stairs at my parents' house, hoping this was all a nightmare. I saw my mom on the phone with documents scattered across the kitchen table. She was reminding her brother where to send Memom for funeral preparations. My uncle was the power of attorney and the only one authorized to arrange affairs with the hospital, funeral home, and the will. Memom had a list of wishes for her funeral to try to make the process easier on the family. Since she spent 17 years working with patients who were at the end of their lives, she saw firsthand the challenges and disagreements if the patient did not have their affairs in order. She had prepared the list, dated November 1, 2013, and provided copies for her children. Titled "Funeral Arrangements When I Depart This Earth," Memom listed the funeral home, burial location next to my grandfather, and details on the "celebration of life." She wanted the celebration to occur at her church, but due to lockdown, this would not be possible. The last three lines were, "Don't be sad. I've had a wonderful life and a loving family. See you later! Love to each of you." I had seen this list before and knew we should respect Memom's wishes.

My uncle said he needed time since this was a lot to take in. The hospital needed to know where to send Memom's body within a few hours of death, and he had not called them yet. Then he started talking about the will and the funeral. Mom mentioned having a celebration of life later in the summer with family, including her brother and sister. Over nearly 30 years, we had only celebrated together one Christmas and Memom's 90th birthday. The chance of having a memorial service later where the entire family would get together was slim. I asked Mom about having a celebration like Memom wanted. Her brother expressed concerns about the safety of people attending a funeral. He said that he would be put at risk and needed to be protected, so he would not be attending. The implication that Mom was putting people in danger by planning a graveside service felt demoralizing.

I only received one day of bereavement from work and decided I would use it for the funeral. With my camera off, I stayed quiet during the work meeting. Anything we talked about felt trivial compared to Memom's death. I had only told two people at work about Memom being in the hospital and wasn't ready to tell anyone she had passed. By the time my meeting was over, my mom had finished speaking with her brother. When I went to the kitchen to see what was happening next, I could see the exhaustion in my mom's face. She seemed shocked her brother accused her of jeopardizing people's health by having an outdoor funeral. It was almost a year into the pandemic, and it felt like every aspect of life was threatened by policies and perceptions. My mom decided to continue planning a funeral as close to what Memom wanted as possible, knowing her brother and sister would not be attending.

During the afternoon of February 17th, I wrote an email to the life enrichment coordinator at Memom's assisted living facility, thanking her for her kindness.

Email to Kyla:

Kyla,

My heart is completely broken with missing Memom already. I was able to see her last night but they only let me in. I told her all the wonderful people in her life who loved her and were praying for her. I held her hand and wanted her to squeeze it one more time but she was too tired. The nurse said Memom knew I was there though.

I love this picture of the both of you. I always felt like you were her guardian angel there and she had a family member who worked there. The special memories you created for me and Memom and our family will always be treasured. I especially love this picture because in the background is also the wonderful moment your husband captured of Memom and Carter. The assisted living facility was her home because of you and Sherri and she loved it. Thank you for everything.

Candace

Memom's funeral was on Wednesday, February 24th; my dad's side of the family was in attendance. Despite the season, the sun was shining and the temperature was in the 60s. A tent and chairs were set up near the tomb where Memom would be placed. Memom was loved by everyone who knew her, and they shared many special memories. Bobby and Mary, Memom's special friends who thought of her as their mother, drove from North Carolina to honor her memory. Her life enrichment coordinator, Kyla, and an aide attended the ceremony as well. My mom asked my sister-in-law to FaceTime the funeral ceremony for family who chose not to attend in person. I didn't know this was planned ahead of time and still couldn't believe the accusation of putting people in danger by gathering outside. Still numb from losing Memom, I sat in the front row and kept to myself. Memom was very religious, and in my room, I kept a framed prayer she gave me a long time ago about living for today. During the service, I read the prayer, hoping I could live up to the meaning of each line.

For Today
By Bishop Phillips Brooks

Give me strength to live another day;
Let me not turn coward before its difficulties
     Or prove recreant to its duties;
Let me not lose faith in other people;
Keep me sweet and sound of heart, in spite of
     Ingratitude, treachery, or meanness;
Preserve me from minding little stings or
     Giving them;
Help me to keep my heart clean, and to live so
     Honestly and fearlessly that no outward

> *Failure can dishearten me or take away the*
> *Joy of conscious integrity;*
> *Open wide the eyes of my soul that I may see*
> *Good in all things;*
> *Grant me this day some new vision of thy truth;*
> *Inspire me with the spirit of joy and gladness;*
> *And make me the cup of strength to suffering*
> *Souls; in the name of the strong Deliverer, our*
> *Only Lord and Savior, Jesus Christ.*

Memom faced many tragic events throughout her life. She could have given up; she could have become bitter. Instead, she persevered. The prayer I read described her outlook perfectly. Her prayer card included "A Nurse's Prayer," since she always loved her profession.

A Nurse's Prayer
By Teri Lynn Thompson, RN

Let me dedicate my life today
To the care of those
Who come my way.

Let me touch each one
With healing hands
And the gentle art
For which I stand.

And when tonight
When the day is done.
Oh, let me rest in peace
If I have helped just one …

Memom requested "Triumphant organ music as I leave the church!!" for her funeral as she didn't want anyone to be sad. My dad brought his guitar, and we sang "Amazing Grace," another song she had requested. Memom knew what she was doing when she chose the music! We started laughing a little when we realized how long the song was. Only my dad can sing well, but we tried to carry a tune. Unexpectedly, I noticed an extra bright floral arrangement with the message "Happy Birthday!" when I was singing. I took it as a sign from Memom not to take life so seriously. The funeral ended with a recording of Johnny and June Carter Cash singing "Will the Circle Be Unbroken?" Memom's mother's side of the family was related to the Cashes; it was a tribute to her family heritage. The guitar music was up-tempo, but the lyrics reflected the sadness we felt.

We honored Memom's request to have pizza after her funeral. Not everyone attended dinner at the local pizzeria, Grotto Pizza, but those who did took time to share their stories and memories of Memom. I tried to focus on the happy times with her, but all I could think about were the unknowns that led to her suffering. I wanted answers.

For about six weeks after losing Memom, I barely left my house. Each day felt meaningless; I blamed myself for losing Memom. I didn't want to be around people since I cried so often. I was relieved that turning on my camera wasn't required for work meetings; I didn't want my crying to draw the attention of others at work.

Eventually, my dad called to check in on me. He said, "You have to live for the living," and explained that Memom wouldn't want us to hold on to the hurt. Easier said than done. I could tell Mom, my best friend, had been holding in a lot of emotions over what Memom went through, too. I slowly began doing something I enjoyed every day. When my mom and I went to a paint night at a local restaurant, we promised ourselves we'd stop the self-blaming and start enjoying life again while still seeking answers from the state investigation.

Records from the Assisted Living Facility
Things We Didn't Know

As medical power of attorney, my mom requested a copy of Memom's records from the assisted living facility while she was still in the hospital, initially thinking we needed to understand what happened to keep Memom safe when she returned to the facility. At that time, we had no idea what the records would show, nor that we would be using the information to gain an understanding of what led to her death. On February 12, 2021, my mom sent a request to the executive director of the facility. No records were sent; we waited a few weeks before trying again. We followed up again in March; the reply we received was also copied to the vice president of operations. At this point, we wanted as much information as possible to hold the facility accountable and knew the records were key to this. The company that owned the assisted living facility had senior living communities across 27 states. We never communicated with anyone in the company above the regional nursing director and didn't understand why a vice president would have to be involved for record release. The only reason we could think of was that they had something to hide. I called a senior social services administrator with the Department of Health & Social Services for help in obtaining the records. Finally, on March 11, 2021, my mom received the records via email, with the company's "legal help" and vice president copied.

Once I started reading the medical records, I couldn't have been more shocked by how long Memom had been suffering. I began to piece together the neglect that led to her painful death. At five feet nine inches, Memom was never very small, but she lost 11 pounds, or almost ten percent of her weight, in eight weeks from September to December 2020. Even more concerning, her quarterly wellness baseline evaluation conducted by the nurse in December 2020 mentioned nothing about her foot wound. In the documents of the evaluation, I found in Memom's writing, "Life is good, hang on!" She was only required to write a single sentence; it could have been anything to show her mental clarity. I tried to understand why Memom would choose that sentence. These words show she valued her life even when she had an infection raging through her body. Each day, I struggled with anger, regret, and sadness over losing Memom. Reading this note reminded me that Memom would not want me to waste my life and was exactly what I needed to see.

The "service notes" document started on May 5, 2020, and included updates from the nurse on any behavioral or physical changes. Podiatrist visits to the facility normally occurred once a month before the pandemic. Memom was seen in her room by the podiatrist on August 19, 2020, with no issues noted. There were no other documented visits from a podiatrist after this date. My mom and I weren't notified of the increased anxiety and number of falls Memom had throughout the month of August. If there was a positive COVID case in the facility, residents would be restricted to their rooms. Social interaction was limited to dining staff dropping off meals in the room three times a day and nursing staff dropping off medicine in the morning and at night. We assumed being confined to a 10-foot by 20-foot room impacted mental health but had no idea how anxious Memom became until we read the records. The notes about Memom's fall in August 2020 stated she used her personal Life Alert button to call 911 and was found lying face down next to her nightstand. The ambulance took Memom to the hospital, and the nurses at the facility spoke with the hospital staff twice during her stay. Memom returned to the facility on September 6, 2020.

On September 25, 2020, the assisted living facility nurse documented that the "resident has redness and shearing to bilateral big toes." My mom wasn't told about this new injury. Based on the records, it was the start of the wound that killed Memom. Brief notes included only that Memom was "seen by" the external nursing agency, without any indication as to what care they were providing or what they found. She was allowed to go to the dentist on October 1, 2020, but no appointments for a podiatrist visit were made. Increased sleepiness and agitation were noted on October 14th. The nurse sent a request for Memom to be checked for a urinary tract infection (UTI) due to these symptoms, but the results came back negative. In the notes, it stated that the "POA," or power of attorney, was notified. We assumed my mom would be the one contacted, as she was listed on the advanced directive as the medical power of attorney. Somehow, the staff confused calling the medical power of attorney, who was my mom, with the power of attorney, who was my mom's brother. I discovered the disconnect in an email exchange with the Regional Director of Care Services on February 11, 2021, after Memom was admitted to the hospital. Infections of all kinds, especially in the elderly, can lead to confusion and agitation. Eight days after the negative test result for the UTI, the nurse noted, "bilateral great toes infected. Bloody sanguine discharge from tips of toes." There was no call to either my mom or her brother about the infection. Only an appointment with an external skilled nursing agency was requested to "evaluate and treat pressure wounds;" there was no appointment for a podiatrist. Antibiotics were administered starting on October 23, 2020. Daily updates included "antibiotics received" and "no complaints" from Memom about pain or discomfort. It didn't surprise me that she made no complaints because she always wanted to avoid the hospital. The antibiotic prescription continued into November, with still no appointment for a doctor to look at her wound. She fell again each day from November 8th through the 11th, with no injury recorded, and the notes indicated "family and doctor notified," but it wasn't clear which family member received notice. Based on record review, it could be assumed that the infection was impacting her ability to walk safely, but no further appointments were made to determine why she was suddenly falling so much.

The wound severity escalated on November 17, 2020, as the "toe was warm to touch, red/ raw, and black eschar." Still no podiatrist appointment. According to the National Pressure Injury Advisory Panel (NPIAP), eschar occurs typically in Stage Three or Four pressure injuries. At this point, Memom's wound was already a higher stage than the assisted living facility was allowed to treat without a waiver, yet they didn't communicate this to my mom. The documentation of the details of Memom's wound shocked me. I thought a trained nurse would've recognized the need to get Memom more care than they were able to provide. Before we had the records, we assumed the staff was too busy to notice Memom's wound, but the records showed the exact opposite situation. The external agency nurse who saw Memom on November 17th told staff at the facility Memom needed to be sent to the emergency room for her foot wound. My mom received a phone call that day from the facility nurse about the foot wound, the first time she was notified. It came as a shock to learn that Memom was going to the emergency room for a wound we had known nothing about until this call. I remember my mom calling me to discuss the nurse's information; we anticipated Memom being transferred to the local hospital. A few hours later, the facility nurse called my mom to tell her they didn't need to send her to the emergency room anymore. At the time, we felt relieved as a hospital stay could've increased Memom's likelihood of catching COVID. Had we understood the severity of the wound, we would have challenged their decision to keep her at the facility. According to state regulations, if facility personnel were aware Memom's wound was above stage 2, they were required to get a waiver with physician and family agreement to allow Memom to stay. This never happened.

The next day, Memom went to her cardiologist for a normal routine appointment. Neither my mom nor I were allowed to attend the appointment with her due to the facility's isolation policies. Her aide accompanied her; since she had seen Memom's toe when she helped her with showers, the aide mentioned the wound to the cardiologist. The cardiologist wrote a note to the facility that Memom needed to see a podiatrist emergently. On November 19, 2020, the external agency nurse visited Memom, and the primary care physician agreed she needed to see her podiatrist. The facility nurse wrote, "resident appeared to be paranoid today." There was no follow-up for this concern.

When I called Memom on the ViewClix, I would often see her sitting in her recliner in a dark room with the blinds shut. I believe a combination of the isolation, darkness, and infection was starting to take over her mind, but I only inferred this from the records. My conversations with Memom were limited as she never really understood how to use the ViewClix device.

The inconsistencies with whom the nurses at the facility contacted were evident in the notes. On November 24, 2020, records stated POA Audrey, who was neither the power of attorney nor the medical power of attorney, was notified of the wound care plan. This happened to also be the only day I was allowed to visit inside the facility, but no one mentioned any issues to me. As Memom sat across the table from me in the bistro room, I saw fear in her eyes, and she barely spoke any words. I could tell I was losing her but didn't know what to do. My plan was to visit more often, and I visited Memom with my mom again on December 1st. This visit should've been our sign to remove Memom from the facility, as two staff members yelled at me on the porch after they discovered I reported the visitation lies to their corporate headquarters. Family visitation was not permitted ever again after that day while Memom was alive. Two days later, my mom requested that

Memom be able to leave her room and walk outside with her aide. The nurse documented she "cannot give that permission but did explain a walking schedule has been implemented for the future." Despite the cardiologist stating Memom needed to see a podiatrist emergently on November 19, 2020, there were no documented visits with podiatry until January 5, 2021—over three months after the first documented concern. At this visit, she returned with no new orders. Once again, my mom and I were not allowed to attend or listen in to the appointment, so we had to rely on Memom or her aide to advocate for better care. We still hadn't seen a picture or video of the wound.

The facility nurse attempted to contact the podiatrist on January 19th with concerns about one of Memom's toes. Two days later, they received a call back with some instructions and scheduled an appointment. Wound care orders included cleaning, applying medicine, and changing the wound dressing. The podiatrist scheduled a follow-up appointment for February 11th. Almost daily after January 21st, Memom was seen by the external agency with "no issues" and no updates to her status. Suddenly, on February 4th, Memom's toe became red and purple, with redness up to her mid-calf. We didn't know this at the time, but the wound was very similar to the one in 2019, over which we decided to cancel the investigation into Memom's neglect. After reading about Memom's long journey of suffering and the knowledge of the injury by medical professionals, I became even more outraged that people could allow a human to endure such pain. There were so many opportunities for someone to step in and get Memom proper treatment. As I finished my review of the medical notes, I made a three-part promise to Memom. I promised to see the investigation through to its completion; I promised to advocate for systemic changes in long-term care facilities; I promised to tell Memom's story whenever I could, to honor her and to help others with aging parents, siblings, grandparents, and friends.

Moving out and journals

We were not allowed to enter the facility to get Memom's belongings out. The director stated that due to COVID-19 protocols, we had to hire a moving company to remove her things. The week after the funeral, my mom's brother scheduled a Zoom call with my mom, her sister, and Memom's aide. It cost $600 to pay the aide for this call and for packing Memom's belongings. My mom didn't have room for all the furniture at her house; the facility sold what was left, with proceeds going to the employee "party fund." A few pieces of furniture were family heirlooms; we made sure to keep those. Memom's beautiful jackets and bows symbolized her vibrant personality; we had them packed up. The movers came a couple of days later to transport the items to my parents' house. My mom didn't tell the moving company representatives the circumstances around Memom's death, but when the movers got to my parents' house, they relayed how shocked they were about what they saw in the facility. The residents' conditions and the treatment the movers received were enough to have one gentleman say he would never have anyone in that facility.

Every day until 2017, Memom recorded her daily activities, including Phillies game details, in a red journal. I never read the journals before she passed away but knew journaling was a part of her daily routine. Memom never complained about the assisted living facility to us, but in her journals, we could get a glimpse of her life there. She wrote about the fun activities the life enrichment coordinator planned and whether she won the Bingo cover-all each day. However, throughout the years, there were instances where no one came to help her with a shower, leaving Memom to use a washcloth for a sponge bath. Showers were already limited to twice a week. Sometimes her help with getting dressed in the morning was late, causing her to rush to breakfast. She decided to stop writing before the lockdowns, but we believed similar patterns of lack of care continued.

Complaint process

I filed a complaint with the Department of Health and Social Services on Friday, February 5, 2021. The night before, I reviewed Memom's electronic record and finally saw a picture of Memom's right foot upon admission to the hospital. With the diagnosis of sepsis and MRSA, I knew the infection had to be severe. I left a voicemail for the supervisor for investigators, and he returned my call within thirty minutes. He agreed to start an investigation immediately and asked me to email him details. In the follow-up email, I included the information I had from the hospital admission and the picture of Memom's wounds. The next week, while Memom was in the hospital, I spoke with an investigator who was already beginning the process to determine what went wrong. At this point, I only focused on corrective actions to make sure Memom was safe when she returned to the assisted living facility. The assigned investigator, Linda, knew Memom from her role at the Hospital for the Chronically Ill. Our discussions focused on the severity of the wound versus what the facility was licensed to do; I was initially happy with the progress. As the week went on and Memom's health significantly declined, I spent less time worrying about the complaint. However, the day after Memom died, I knew a complaint investigation needed to be completed to prevent others from suffering the same outcome.

Email to Investigator on February 17, 2021

Linda,

My grandmother, Mary Claudia Jones-Barthelmeh passed away last night due to her foot infection. Her records from the hospital should be available. I finally convinced the hospital on Monday to not let her suffer in pain. When I visited Saturday she was thrashing around and it was one of the worst things I've ever seen. Sunday we were told she had a few hours so when she was stable on Monday I asked for morphine since nothing had been given to her since 3 pm Sunday. Her nurse yesterday said she was healthy, but the infection got her. I would like the fullest investigation possible into the terrible events that led to this.

Thank you,

Candace Esham

Communication with Linda lessened as time went on. We exchanged a few emails in March but nothing after that. Complaints can be classified as "immediate jeopardy" if "noncompliance has placed the health and safety of recipients in its care at risk for serious injury, serious harm, serious impairment, or death," according to CMS. Immediate jeopardy events are supposed to be investigated quickly to protect individuals from the same neglect. I believed Memom's death could have been prevented, and others would be harmed if actions weren't taken. We also decided to interview several lawyers to investigate Memom's death as an option to hold the facility accountable. One of the lawyers who specialized in elder care law told me, "If we held every facility accountable for neglect, there would be none open, and we need them." Obviously, I chose not to move forward with this attorney, but it was disheartening to hear from someone who spends their career with families experiencing elder neglect stating how broken the system is. The second attorney we contacted agreed to look into our case as long as we could get the records and if the state completed an investigation. Throughout the summer of 2021, my mother and I reached out to several legislators to help push the state investigation, but there was no sign of progress.

On Monday, October 11, 2021, I received a call from the state health department regarding the investigation of Memom's neglect. The investigator said she found no issues and that they were closing the case. I described the timeline of events leading up to Memom's hospital admission based on the medical records provided by the facility. She questioned how I knew these dates, and I was shocked to learn she hadn't requested any medical records. Only interviews with the staff at the assisted living facility were conducted to lead to the conclusion that nothing wrong had happened. One of the comments from the nurses at the assisted living facility was that Memom was under hospice care and that is why they did not seek further treatment. We were never asked about hospice care during the lockdown. We never signed any waivers for Memom to stay in the assisted living facility with a wound requiring care beyond that which their license covered. According to Delaware Code Title 16 Division of Health Care Quality for Assisted Living Facilities Section 5.9, "an assisted living facility shall not admit, provide services to, or permit the provision of services to individuals who, as established by the resident assessment, have developed stage three or four skin ulcers." The regulations allow residents who are under the care of a hospice program licensed by the department to remain in an assisted living facility with written assurance that all of the resident's needs will be met without placing other residents at risk. The investigators never confirmed the paperwork and only took the word of the facility. Even though I was the family member who filed the complaint, when I brought up my concerns about the false information, the investigator requested to speak to my mom as the medical power of attorney. The investigator called my mom and decided to reopen the case based on the information provided. We had already waited months and didn't know the timeline for the follow-up.

On Friday, October 15, 2021, I went to pick up the medical records from the lawyer we were considering using. I told the receptionist that I was still pursuing justice and that I was going to make sure the nurses involved had another employment option. The receptionist said, "Oh, why would you want that?" I was confused by her comment and asked what she meant. She replied, "Well, I don't want them as my nurse." I clarified I didn't want them to be nurses anywhere to do more harm. It amazed me that someone could accept that it is okay for a negligent nurse to be employed around the elderly, who make up one of the most vulnerable populations, but not okay for the general population, who likely would be able to advocate for themselves. Since we didn't have the complaint investigation, we decided not to pursue using this lawyer at the time. The likelihood of the lawyer proving neglect without the support of the state would have been too challenging; we did not want to waste money or time.

Finally, on November 19, 2021, investigators visited the assisted living facility to interview staff, perform observations, and review clinical records. At this point, our case had been escalated to the Compliance Nurse Supervisor with the state. Even though the survey was completed, the state and the assisted living facility management negotiated back and forth several times before agreeing on the plan for correction. Families are not included in any part of the investigation, including the interview process. Negotiations occur only between the facility administrators and the state investigators. When deficiencies are found, the administrator must identify actions to address the root cause of the deficiency, also known as the plan for correction. We didn't receive the report until February 22, 2022, after I spoke about the delay in the report at the state Joint Finance Committee, where the Secretary of Health & Social Services was present. The 32-page survey included a sample of 5 residents out of the 60 at the facility. On the first page in the column titled "administrator's plan for correction of deficiencies," there was an odd disclosure:

"Submission of this response and Plan of Correction is NOT a legal admission that a deficiency exists or that this Statement of Deficiencies was correctly cited and is also NOT to be construed as an admission against interest by the residence, or any employees, agents, or other individuals who drafted or may be discussed in the response or Plan of Correction. In addition, preparation and submission of this Plan of Correction does NOT constitute an admission or agreement of any kind by the facility of the truth of any facts alleged or the correctness of any conclusions set forth in this allegation by the survey agency."

It seemed contradictory for the state to find deficiencies, yet this statement implied the facility did not agree. Since the vice president of the company and the legal department were already copied on other emails to my mom, I should have anticipated a lack of admission of fault. Later, after sharing the report with others, I would learn no one had seen this kind of statement on a report. As I continued reading, I had mixed feelings of anger, validation, and sadness.

To protect resident confidentiality, names are not used in the report, and residents are assigned numbers. However, based on the information, I could tell Memom was "R1." Confirming what I already knew, the facility was not allowed to treat a resident with a stage 3 or 4 pressure ulcer without a waiver from the family. Memom's wound on her left great toe was "unstageable" on October 29, 2020, and a new stage 2 pressure ulcer developed on her right great toe. "Unstageable" means the dead tissue, black in appearance, completely covers the wound. Despite the thorough notes from the facility, the interviews claimed there was a lack of awareness of the wound by the care service manager. The root cause determined the Third-Party Provider policy and charting form were not utilized. I didn't understand how the facility nurse could bring in a home health care agency without notifying the care services manager. Especially when visitation was limited during the lockdown, wouldn't staff question who was coming into the building and which residents they were seeing?

Also, the facility failed to request a resident-specific waiver. The waiver includes multiple pieces of information to be completed by a physician, including details on how staff will provide care, why denial of the waiver would impose a substantial hardship for the resident, why the waiver will not adversely affect the resident, and the duration of the waiver, not to exceed 90 days. After Memom's fall in August 2020, the nurse at the facility was supposed to update the "uniform assessment instrument," which is used to determine the needs of the resident and eligibility for an assisted living facility. Depending on the assessment, a higher level of care could have been needed. A common theme throughout the deficiencies was inadequate communication and a misunderstanding of policies or procedures. Audits and training were assigned as plans of correction.

Another resident, "R3," was documented to have similar deficiencies in care, with the service agreement not being updated when their condition changed. Two out of the five resident files reviewed showed a pattern of staff not understanding policies to ensure the safety of residents. The number of resident records surveyed was not expanded, despite what I consider a high rate of issues. Surveys don't include what happened to the residents who were subject to the neglect, and I wondered if the other resident survived. It wasn't clear if the staff involved had received initial or continuing education on the policies they failed to follow. Since I was trained in root cause analysis for my engineering roles, I knew the real root cause and corrective actions should've gone deeper. While there was a lot of information in the report, I didn't know what would've prevented the staff from failing to follow procedures. Was the training never done, not done with enough frequency, or was it not effective? At this point, I didn't push for any further clarification on the report; I had to be satisfied that the investigation identified the failure of staff to follow regulations.

Forgiveness

Not only did I lose my Memom in this horrible tragedy, but our extended family also changed too. My mom's brother lives in Florida, and her sister lives in Colorado. We were the only family Memom had in Delaware and made decisions on care for Memom. During the early part of the pandemic, we were hopeful that this lockdown would only last a couple of weeks and that life could go back to normal. Florida's handling of the pandemic was vastly different from Delaware's management. Families were allowed to see loved ones in facilities after a couple of months, and isolation was limited in Florida.

In early December, after my mom and I were treated rudely by the staff, my mom told her brother about the incident. She expressed concern about other options for Memom's care. I was not a part of the conversation, but my mom felt like he implied we were partly to blame in the confrontation. When my mom asked her brother and sister about bringing Memom to my parents' house for Christmas, they both feared Memom would catch COVID-19. It is hard to believe that someone thought that a home where people cared about Memom more than anyone else and had limited people coming in and out compared to the facility would endanger Memom. However, we didn't even get to see her on Christmas through a window. I didn't want to keep Memom there but couldn't have her at my house due to not having a first-floor bedroom. Despite the facility staff claiming that their protocols protected residents, around Christmas 2020, there was a COVID-19 outbreak at the assisted living facility. Twenty-six staff members tested positive, and eight residents died from COVID-19.

Since the discussion in January 2021, in which I proposed moving Memom to Florida, I had not spoken to my mom's brother. The first weekend Memom was in the hospital, I overheard my mom on a call with her brother and sister. We had yet to be able to communicate with Memom since the nurses had not charged the iPad. Her brother got approval from the hospital nurse to visit Memom but was nervous about flying due to worrying about getting sick. I couldn't understand how he got any preference over my mom and me since we were local. He didn't end up coming, and we didn't get to see her that weekend either.

My brother had a small wedding ceremony for immediate family in November 2020. His big wedding ceremony was held in June 2021. My aunt flew in from Colorado, and my uncle, his wife, and daughter flew in from Florida. It was the first time I had seen them in years and the first opportunity I had to speak to them since Memom's death. I don't believe I had healed enough from what happened to Memom. I still held on to a lot of anger, guilt, and blame. My health was declining due to chronic migraine and facial pain exacerbated by stress. Every night, I had nightmares of Memom screaming in pain, and every morning, I woke up in pain. I continually replayed what I could have done differently to reduce her suffering or prevent her death. Trauma and stress impacted my nervous system function, causing excruciating pain to the point of nausea and blacking out. I didn't want my mom to feel guilty about choosing for Memom to stay in the facility and held in a lot of guilt. Years after Memom passed, with lots of treatments and stress management techniques, I was able to have pain-free days with some consistency.

I regret not speaking to my mom's family at what was one of the happiest days of my brother's life. It took me several months to realize that forgiveness was key to lifting the burden and weight of the anger and grief. Forgiveness can't change the past, but there was a good chance that it would make my future better.

Letter I mailed to my uncle January 2022:

I wanted to let you know that I forgive you. I forgive you for yelling that Memom would be dead if she lived in Florida during the pandemic and hanging up on me. I forgive you for not apologizing for that either. I forgive you for not wanting Mom to have a funeral and for saying you protected her from the stress of seeing your dad on his last day alive.

I wanted to tell you about some things you may not know about what Memom suffered through and how strong she is. I know you miss her dearly as do I. I have been reading through Memom's journals as well as the medical records and working every week to seek justice for what was done to her. Even before the pandemic she struggled to get good care at the assisted living but never complained. When she had shingles, which I found not the nurses, frequently no one would come to put cream on her back and she would try to get through the night. This lack of care escalated when Mom and I were locked out of the facility. The nurses documented her foot wound starting September of 2020 but did not let us know of the situation until a couple months later. They delayed podiatrist care. I truly believed they thought of her as old and did not want to pursue the right care plan. The quote mom sent you, "Life is good, hang on!" is from Memom's medical records. She would get evaluated every 3 months and have to write a sentence to show mental clarity. That was her sentence during her last evaluation in December 2020. I had pored over the medical records but did not find that until a couple months ago. My friends who are nurses have reviewed the records and stated Memom had to have been in incredible pain during the time leading up to her death. When the wound care nurse wanted to send Memom to the hospital in November and Melinda canceled it my friend could tell from the notes that her toe was dead then. It makes me sick the level of detail in the records and lack of sense of urgency. When she went to the hospital, I truly thought an amputation would be the most severe consequence.

I have been working on advocacy with the Delaware Nursing Home quality commission since January of 2021. We are not the only family who has had a loved one suffer unnecessarily but most families are burnt out by the loss of their loved one and don't pursue advocacy. I know Memom would want me to keep pushing for change to help people. I have been sick with anger and hurt and disbelief that people who are in the profession to provide medical care could document her wound and basically shut the door on her. I need to work on forgiveness to not carry that burden anymore for my own health. I thought I would start with you but it will take a long time before I forgive the nurses. I wanted to share a glimpse of what Memom went through. I am documenting more but it is taking time to process.

I miss Memom every day and forget that I can't call her or see her anymore. Locking up the elderly and letting them suffer is going to be looked at as elder genocide. I am going to keep sharing her story of her love of life and how time was stolen from her.

Hope you had a good Christmas and hope this letter helps explain how I have been feeling this year.

Candace

I never heard anything from my mom's brother but know he received the letter. My mom texted him about it, and he said he read it. It disappointed me that he did not have the courage to have a discussion or reach out to me, but I had a sense of peace knowing I tried.

Media after the hospitalization

On February 10th, the reporter from the Delaware State News reached out to check if Memom received her second dose as planned on February 4th. Initial email exchanges started on January 22, 2021, before Memom was hospitalized. In the midst of dealing with the hospitalization and getting through each day, I didn't update the reporter until he sent the email. Hopeful that Memom would survive the wound, I emailed him back late in the evening of February 10th and included the picture of her foot wound.

Hey Tim,

Thank you so much for checking in on me and my family. I did see the announcement yesterday regarding the update for second doses for those who received it at DMV events. I saw Georgetown DMV recipients would have to drive to Dover Downs. My mom has been looking at the Walgreens website multiple times a day and it always says no appointments available. We haven't been able to get my grandmother into Walgreens online (she doesn't remember her security question answers and we were on hold for 45 minutes today before giving up). My mom is going to call the pharmacy at Walgreens and see if they can help her in store. I attended the town hall coffee chat with Kevin Hensley yesterday and a lot of other residents have issues getting registered. You can find a replay of the session on his Facebook page. I start speaking 9 minutes in.

As far as my grandmother in the assisted living, she received her second dose last Thursday. We were called Thursday morning and told my grandmother needed to be taken to the hospital for wounds on her feet but they wanted to wait till after she got the vaccine. I attached the picture of what her foot looked like upon arrival to the hospital. I fully believe because my family and I have been isolated and not able to be involved in her care that this resulted in her going to the hospital with sepsis and MRSA. We were told in November she had wounds on her foot but have been told things were getting better. My mother, who is medical POA, requested copies of the notes last Friday but has not received a release form or a call back. My grandmother's second toe fell off last night. She is still in the hospital and we are planning what our options are. We are able to have one person FaceTime her once a day, if they charged the iPad. The governor of Florida recognized the neglect and abuse going on in nursing homes and assisted livings and that is why he modified the visitation policy for families. According to AARP.org dashboard (AARP dashboard), Florida has the lowest resident death ratio and positive case rate. So if we have a model where families are allowed to be involved in the care, quality of life, and safety of their loved ones with the lowest issue with COVID, why has Delaware done NOTHING. Representative Kevin Hensley has spoken to the governor about his concerns regarding long term care facilities but nothing has been done. I am not sure I will forgive myself for not demanding to know what was going on with different people or something to have prevented this.

As a side note, when I was able to FaceTime my grandmother on Monday, we left it on for awhile and I was able to watch her enjoy the Delaware State News, which she reads daily. I know vaccine coverage is a huge priority but the neglect going on in nursing homes is terrifying.

Talk to you soon hopefully.
Candace

Tim returned my email the next day, stating there was still interest in a story on long-term care. I thanked him and passed along information I learned from the nurse at the assisted living facility: residents who returned to the facility from the hospital were no longer being tested for COVID before coming back into the facility. It was unclear how the decision was made. The day after Memom passed away, I emailed, explaining how devastating losing Memom was to my family. Even though Memom was gone, I still believed press coverage of the systemic issues in the long-term care industry would drive changes and prevent others from suffering neglect.

Tim,

I just wanted to give you an update. I heard you ask questions at the press conference yesterday and I am thankful for the ones you asked. I appreciate your dedication. My Memom passed away last night due to infection from her foot. I was the only one allowed to see her yesterday. I am heartbroken and will continue advocating so others do not have to suffer like she did. I have the state investigating them due to the wound. On a positive note, my mother was able to get signed up for her second dose on Monday. We got her scheduled this morning for the Dover event. I asked other family to help my other grandmother get signed up since I am helping with the funeral arrangements.

Thanks,

Candace

On March 5, 2021, Tim confirmed a series of articles would be published over several days marking the one-year anniversary of the first positive COVID case, including the story on long-term care facilities. I provided official comments to support the story but unfortunately learned on March 14th that the story was pushed back due to new guidance on visitation from the Centers for Medicare and Medicaid Services. Requests from Tim for additional information came every couple of weeks, along with more notifications of delays on the story. Finally, on June 24, 2021, Tim explained his goal of finishing the story by the 4th of July. I wrote back with hopes that the story would be published soon and never heard back after my June 28, 2021, email. A story wasn't published with the *Delaware State News*, and I waited a few weeks before starting over in my quest to find a journalist. In March 2023, the journalist took a role as Deputy Director of Communications for the Delaware Department of Health and Social Services.

Part 2

Advocacy On My Own

Throughout the process of the state complaint investigation and pursuit of media attention, I began trying to influence legislators to improve long-term care policies. My professional career as an engineer included training on root cause analysis, benchmarking best practices, and implementing programs to reduce the risk of system failures. I had experience in the nuclear power industry, medical device manufacturing, project management in a major hospital system, and was currently working in chemical manufacturing. Each of these industries relied on mitigating errors to ensure safety and quality were a priority. In my mind, I thought if I researched data as well as identified root causes and corrective actions, stakeholders involved in long-term care would be willing to listen. One benefit of the lockdown was that state government meetings started to offer virtual options, allowing the public better access to attend meetings.

Delaware is only 96 miles long, varying from 9 to 35 miles in width. Dover, the state capital, is in the center of the state and is no more than 90 minutes from any part of the state. Despite the convenience of the location of the capital, when meetings were only held in person, working citizens had limited ability to attend. I was working remotely and could move around my schedule to accommodate attending a meeting. While I knew about developing strategies for change, I wasn't very familiar with the legislative process to create or modify regulations. The Delaware General Assembly has 21 senators and 41 representatives. With a state population of approximately one million people, each representative has about 24,000 constituents. My goal was to attend as many meetings as I could to provide public comment, try to convince my local legislator to help sponsor some bills, and have Memom's story on the front page of a newspaper.

Interactions with my State Representative

The state legislature's purposes are to create laws, approve the budget for state government, and provide priorities for government agencies, including their policies and budgets. In my district, the representative held monthly meetings with constituents and generally was more accessible than my senator. I knew that without a representative or senator sponsoring changes to regulations, nothing would improve. Leading up to Memom's death, I attempted to convince state agencies that their policy decisions were negatively impacting the elderly. This only led to frustration and the realization that they get their direction from elected officials. I sent the first email to my representative the day after Memom was admitted to the hospital. In his January town hall, I voiced my concerns but hadn't heard anything since then.

I emailed Representative Hensley on the afternoon of Friday, February 5th.

Good afternoon Kevin,

I am reaching out because our elderly who are in nursing homes, long term care facilities, and assisted living are being neglected. Specifically, my grandmother has been dealing with wounds on her right foot for weeks now due to being confined to her room majority of the day. Her exercise previously has been walking to the dining room 3 times a day and most days she has not been allowed to even leave her room. She is now in the hospital with sepsis and a potential bone infection. I have reached out to the facility, reached out to the state of Delaware, and am filing a complaint but preventing families from being able to check on their loved ones is dangerous. Florida has the lowest death rate in the U.S in nursing homes according to AARP (https://www.aarp.org/ppi/issues/caregiving/info-2020/nursing-home-covid-dashboard.html) and has provided a safe way for families to see their loved ones because their governor recognized the neglect happening.

Please help me work on a safe way to have families ensure our loved ones are safe and cared for. I can be reached via email or cell phone.

Thanks,

Candace

Email sent to Kevin Hensley February 19, 2021

Kevin,

I hope you are well. I wanted to let you know I filed a complaint with the board of health over my Memom's lack of care at the assisted living facility. On February 2, 2021, Memom was admitted to Kent General with sepsis and MRSA. I requested the medical records from the assisted living facility and on January 19th, the nursing staff documented tunneling of the foot and pustulate coming out. My mother, who is medical power of attorney, was never notified. No doctor was called and no additional treatment given. She passed away the night of 2/16. The ICU nurse told me her body was so strong and the foot infection caused this.

This is what happens when families are not allowed to be involved in the care and well-being of their loved ones. We did not know my mother had full authority to override my uncle until we spoke with the lawyer on January 25th. We had a plan to try to get to see her but didn't act fast enough. When my mother called my other grandmother to let her know of Memom's passing she cried and said please don't let something like this happen to me. It is hard to put into words how heartbroken I am that Memom was treated this way. I am hoping the state decision makers look to more success-ful models like Florida for care of the elderly.

Thanks,

Candace

Response from Kevin on February 22, 2021

Hi Candace,

Thank you very much for keeping me up to date -- I truly appreci-ate it and am so very sorry for your loss. I am praying for you and your family.

Please keep me posted on the status of the complaint -- this is absolutely unacceptable and I am certainly willing to get involved if you need me.

Thanks,

Kevin

Response to Kevin on February 22, 2021

Hi Kevin,

Thank you so much for getting back to me, as always, and for the prayers. My family and I truly appreciate it. We are getting the death certificate to the state investigators this week and the lead investigator has been very thorough so far. She used to be a wound care nurse and I couldn't ask for a better person to look into things to hopefully prevent this from happening to someone else. I will keep you posted.

Also, on Friday I spoke with Margaret Bailey, the executive director of the Delaware Nursing Home Residents Quality Assurance Commission. She mentioned the commission is up for evaluation for whether it should receive state funding. I wrote a testimony on behalf of support for the Commission tonight but would appreciate your support on continuing funding for them (if not expanding). DNHRQAC's mission is to monitor Delaware's quality assurance system for nursing home residents in both privately operated and state operated facilities so that complaints of abuse, neglect mistreatment, financial exploitation and other complaints are responded to in a timely manner so as to ensure the health and safety of nursing home residents. I fully believe this is necessary to protect our residents in these facilities.

Thank you again for your support. I'm very thankful you are my representative.

Thanks,

Candace

Joint Finance Committee Meeting February 2021

Legislative session in Delaware is held from January to June each year. This is the only time bills can be developed to change laws, which drive state priorities and new laws. One of the key aspects of the session is writing the annual appropriations, or operating budget. In fact, a balanced budget bill is the only constitutionally required bill for each session. A 12-member Joint Finance Committee, comprised of six members of the Senate Finance Committee and six members of the House Appropriations Committee, conducts public hearings on state agency budget requests based on the Governor's Recommended Budget. Each member of the public in attendance is allowed two minutes to speak. Since I repeatedly heard about resource and financial constraints from the Division of Health Care Quality, I assumed the Joint Finance Committee would be a good place to ask for more funding.

The Joint Finance Committee Hearing for the Fiscal Year 2022 budget for the Division of Health and Social Services was held virtually via Zoom on February 23, 2021. With lockdown protocols still in effect, state legislators could not convene in person. Each fiscal year, the Governor develops a proposed budget for state spending. All line items greater than $100,000 are reviewed by this committee, and recommended adjustments are made based on input from members of the committee. State legislative meetings still were mostly held remotely due to a continued state of emergency order. During the discussion portion of the meeting, Representative Ruth Briggs King expressed concern around the quality assessments of long-term care facilities, stating around 86% of COVID deaths occurred in residents of these facilities. She stated that only two or three surveyors from the state were available to inspect the 80+ licensed facilities in Delaware. Lack of visitation ability for families of residents in long-term care facilities contributed to the lack of comfort level with the oversight. The secretary of the division attributed inspector staffing issues to the extra training required for investigations. Infection prevention inspections were prioritized over standard surveys that ensure safety and quality of other aspects of care.

Since this was my first time listening to and commenting on the Joint Finance Committee, I prepared a written statement to read to ensure I stayed under my two-minute time allotment. Over ninety minutes passed since the start of the meeting, and I didn't know before the meeting if my comments would be new or if they would resonate with some of the legislators. A few other members of the public spoke before me regarding concerns with the lack of services currently available for those with substance abuse issues in recovery, issues with grants to primary care providers, and problems with contractual rates between government and non-profits. I supported the continued funding of the Delaware Nursing Home Residents Quality Assurance Commission (DNHRQAC). Describing Memom's foot wound timeline, my voice wavered, and I began crying when I announced the date Memom died. Watching the two-minute timer tick down, I quickly pulled myself back together to finish my thoughts. I emphasized the importance of oversight to ensure the health and safety of long-term care facilities. No other members of the public commented after me. Representative Kim Williams expressed sympathy for my loss and mentioned she served on DNHRQAC. Another senator followed, redirecting the conversation back to budget line items. The call lasted a few more minutes and ended with a break for lunch. It felt crushing to be limited to describing the pain of losing Memom to two minutes and then to only have one legislator respond. I ended the Zoom call with emotions of anger and disbelief at how callous people who represent the welfare of constituents with regulations could be. How could they not react to a horrific tragedy? Unsure of any other path forward, I wrote Representative Williams a thank-you email the next day.

Email to Representative Kim Williams

Good morning Representative Williams,

I wanted to thank you for the kind words after I spoke about my Memom yesterday on the Joint Finance Committee call. I am completely heartbroken over how it all happened but I know my Memom would want me to continue to be an advocate for the elderly. She saw an advertisement in the movies for free nursing school at Emory University if she agreed to be a cadet nurse in WWII. She met my grandfather who was a pilot in the Air Force and traveled the world with him. When they settled at the Dover Air Force base for retirement, Memom retook her nursing exams at the age of 50. She worked at the Hospital for the Chronically Ill until she retired at 68.

Nursing was a passion for my Memom. Even though I am an engineer I would always love listening to the stories about her dear patients. As I mentioned yesterday, it is unfortunate what happened to my grandmother but she would want me to share her story to help others. I appreciate the work you do for the elderly and look forward to working with Margaret more as well. I would like to see an Elder Caucus established for the state of Delaware. Please let me know if I can do anything to support this.

Thank you again for your support. I look forward to speaking again sometime.

Thanks,

Candace Esham

Delaware Nursing Home Residents
Quality Assurance Commission

I decided to join the Delaware Nursing Home Residents Quality Assurance Commission meetings to advocate for changes. The next quarterly meeting occurred on March 16, 2021. Since the state employee who would lead the meeting called me back on a Sunday, I was hopeful I had finally found a group where people recognized the severity of issues and the need to act. Members included representatives from the long-term care industry, public advocates, legislators, and physicians. The meeting began with a lengthy discussion about adult guardianship, which is needed primarily for individuals with dementia, traumatic brain injury, autism, or other cognitive issues who have no other alternatives to care management. I wasn't familiar with this process, so I waited for an opportunity to speak about my concerns regarding neglect in assisted living facilities. According to meeting minutes, the Director of the Division of Health Care Quality usually joined the meeting to discuss long-term care facility surveys and complaints. Due to technical difficulties, she was not able to join the Zoom call. Next, an update on the status of the long-term care ombudsman program: The long-term care ombudsman advocates for residents who live in long-term care facilities, including investigating and resolving complaints. Since ombudsmen provide a key voice for residents, it troubled me that no ombudsmen had been allowed in person at any facility in the entire state since December 1, 2020. Video meetings or telephone calls were options; with only 75 total interactions in almost four months for the entire state, however, I believed a lot of residents were essentially voiceless. Another commission member echoed my thoughts, but no actions were taken to address the concern.

The Executive Director, Margaret Bailey, shared sobering statistics regarding the number of deaths due to COVID. As of March 14, 2021, there were a total of 1,511 deaths in Delaware attributed to COVID. Of those who had died, 719, or almost forty-eight percent, were long-term care facility residents. Despite the strict visitation guidelines enforced by facilities and state officials, outbreaks occurred in these facilities. On March 10, 2021, the Centers for Medicaid and Medical Assistance (CMS), in collaboration with the Centers for Disease Control and Prevention (CDC), issued new guidance for expanded visitation options in nursing homes. This included stating that facilities should always allow responsible indoor visitations for all residents, with only a couple of scenarios limiting visitation. These scenarios included limitations for unvaccinated residents, if the COVID county positivity rate is greater than 10 percent and less than 70 percent of residents in the facility are fully vaccinated, residents who tested positive for COVID, and residents in quarantine. The Delaware Division of Health and Social Services adopted the new federal guidelines on March 26, 2021. Visits, both indoor and outdoor, had been restricted since December 2020.

A reference was made to a question in the Joint Finance Committee Budget hearing in the previous month regarding long-term care facility surveys. The state auditor stated she provided a response but did not elaborate on the details. Despite the mission of the commission to monitor Delaware's quality assurance system for nursing home residents, it seemed as if the commission lacked the details to understand the systemic issues inflicting harm on residents. I initially attributed the minimal data about complaints and survey findings to the inability of the director of the Division of Health Care Quality to join the call. Since this was my first time attending, I only listened to the meeting and didn't contribute to the conversation. Still hopeful that the commission was the right forum to advocate for policy changes, I kept attending the quarterly meetings.

The next meeting, May 18, 2021, hosted more members of the public and state representatives, including the secretary of the Division of Health and Social Services, several staff in the Division of Health Care Quality (DHCQ), and the Division of Services for Aging Adults with Physical Disabilities. Updates were provided by each of the departments, including that since January 1, 2021, DHCQ had already received 1,415 complaints. I reflected on the previous meeting's report, where the ombudsman program for the entire state only completed 75 interactions from December 2020 to March 2021, and the state had received almost 19 times the number of complaints within a four-month span. I wondered how there could be such a huge difference between the two numbers. Since March 1, 2021, the ombudsmen were allowed to resume in-person visits, but I worried about all the residents who did not have an advocate during the restricted time. According to a meeting attendee, posters about how to contact the ombudsman for a virtual visit were displayed in a few designated common areas, but residents were often restricted to their rooms, leaving them with no knowledge of how to reach help. The timeline for investigating the significant volume of complaints was unclear, which meant behaviors leading to the complaint could potentially continue. This was the first time I became aware of how many other loved ones experienced neglect and submitted a complaint. At the end of the meeting, outraged at the lack of urgency to investigate the complaints, I shared Memom's story of suffering for months with a foot wound that led to a painful death. An outcome of the investigation process is a corrective action plan to prevent a similar occurrence. Without completing it in a timely manner, other residents in Memom's assisted living facility were vulnerable to harm. The long-term care ombudsman program committed to assist me in the process because I spoke up. They ultimately did not fulfill their commitment.

During my third meeting in July 2021, I began to realize the intent of the agenda was to provide updates but not conduct problem-solving. Each meeting, a few concerns would be discussed, but no action plan or subcommittee had been created to resolve the issues. I became more vocal about policy changes that could be enacted to institute sustainable improvements to current system failures. Specifically, when the ombudsman program was mentioned again, I asked how regulations could ensure ombudsmen would be considered essential personnel with ongoing access to facilities. The executive director stated she suggested this a few years ago, but nothing was done. A note was taken to consider exploring this requirement, but there was no real commitment to follow up. My fear of delay in complaint investigations was validated as only 43 complaints were investigated from March 2021 to July 2021. With a backlog of over 1,400 complaints reported in March, it would take eight years to complete investigations at this rate, assuming no new submissions. Complaints regarding the deaths of residents were supposed to receive the highest priority, but Memom's complaint had still not been investigated more than five months after her passing. In the six annual surveys completed, abuse and neglect rose to the top five citations. It seemed obvious to me that neglect in the facilities would continue until administrators were held accountable. Less obvious was what would need to happen to create the urgency for change. Civil Monetary Penalties—fines imposed on a facility for violations—could be used by various organizations, including long-term care facilities, if the funds were to be used to improve the quality of care or quality of life of residents residing in federally certified nursing homes. No facilities applied for the funds in 2020, leading me to believe that no facilities prioritized quality improvement projects. In other meetings, I heard industry representatives describe the financial troubles facilities faced during the pandemic, so I silently questioned why facilities wouldn't apply for available money if they were supposedly focused on quality care.

I knew nothing I could do would lessen Memom's suffering, and I wanted my family's story to be enough to convince state officials to do a better job with oversight. Again, I shared Memom's story and my family's unfruitful quest for answers five months after her passing. I joined calls in September 2021, November 2021, January 2022, and March 2022 before realizing each call resulted in data reports without any solutions. Learning how pervasive and long-standing issues with care at assisted living facilities were, I knew it would take more than just me attending meetings to make changes. As an engineer who specializes in regulations and performance improvement, I had never seen solutions developed for complex, widespread problems come out of simply having a meeting. Almost a year and a half into my advocacy journey, I felt no closer to finding a group that knew how to problem-solve and only became aware of more problems and excuses. Juggling a full-time job, attending meetings, and trying to get media attention started to take a toll on my mental and physical health. Each day I felt desperate to give Memom's suffering a purpose. State officials whose jobs were to enforce quality and accountability for long-term care facilities seemed exasperated by the volume of issues. Each call had only a couple of public members join, and I was usually the only one who spoke up. Knowing there were well over 1,000 complaints in the backlog, I wondered whether the families who filed them had lost faith in resolution. I maintained my commitment to finding a journalist who could help me spread the word about the systemic issues and traumatic stories from residents at facilities in hopes of gaining legislators' attention.

Joint Finance Committee Hearings February 2022

At the time of the Joint Finance Committee Hearings for DHSS and DHCQ in 2022, Mom and I were still desperately trying to get answers from the state about what happened to Memom. We knew the assisted living facility was found negligent in caring for Memom but had no access to the details or the plan of correction determined to protect current and future residents. The manager of the investigation department emailed my mom on January 5, 2022, alerting her that the investigation was complete. Requiring the family to then relentlessly email and call for the report, even though it was available for public records, added to the stress of the broken process. We learned that while the investigation was completed in November 2021, the facility and Division of Health Care Quality had not yet agreed upon the plan of correction. Since legislators would not return our emails or phone calls regarding the investigation, the only platform I had for help was the Joint Finance Committee Hearing's public comment period. One legislator in Dover did reply and helped push for the completion of the investigation as well.

The hearing meetings were scheduled for Tuesday, February 22nd, and Wednesday, February 23rd. I decided to speak on the first day, after the overall DHSS presentation, in hopes my comments would provide the legislators with questions for the DHCQ meeting. Public comment always follows the legislator question period, and the next topic is brought up or the meeting moves on. In my experience, the people who take the time to listen to the meeting in hopes of getting two minutes to speak their thoughts on the topic have the keenest insight into the most details regarding the subject. If legislators followed up with questions after the public comment as well, it would give them real-world examples of where the system is broken. Secretary Molly Magarik presented the budget details, accomplishments, and challenges, including the COVID-19 response. Since the department covers all aspects of health, questions can vary. A significant portion of the discussion was regarding visually impaired students and challenges with services for them. Infant mortality and prenatal care were discussed for almost 45 minutes. Hospitals restricted doulas, advocates for mothers, during the pandemic; this generated almost 30 minutes of discussion. Five hundred people in the state were waiting for Section 8 housing or low-income housing, and legislators asked what the state could do to help them more, including vetting reputable hotel owners. The DHSS employee vacancy rate and low salaries took up several minutes of the discussion as well.

There were no questions asked about care for seniors in the community or in institutions. While adequate care for all citizens is important, a glaring oversight was not discussing the largest population of vulnerable people: seniors in our state, specifically in long-term care facilities. In both the overview and financial presentation, COVID-19 impacts were discussed. This included discussion on significant taxpayer funds to support long-term care facilities, but no attention was given to the quality-of-care challenges. Death and neglect in long-term care were prevalent, but in this meeting, they seemed non-existent. My own representative was a member of the Joint Finance Committee, knew we were struggling to get the investigation results, and did not advocate for the elderly. I spoke the following:

Good morning, my name is Candace Esham and I am speaking today just as I did last year to provide support for additional FTEs for the Delaware Nursing home residents quality assurance commission. On February 16, 2021, my grandmother died from sepsis and MRSA from a foot infection that started 5 months prior in an assisted living. It has been 382 days since I filed the complaint and my family still does not have the report. 334 days after I submitted the complaint we were notified neglect was confirmed by the state of Delaware in regards to my grandmother and also another resident but the assisted living has failed to put forward an acceptable corrective action plan three times. Would you accept this response if your child or dog were treated this way and no actions were taken over a year later? Unfortunately, this delay is not just due to pandemic issues as Delaware is one of 10 states that did not meet CMS' performance threshold for timeliness for eight consecutive years from 2011 to 2018. The commission has also challenged the number of vacancies in the Delaware healthcare quality division, which performs investigations. Recently, I came across 30 pages of public comment asking for expansion of the commission. This can be found in the joint legislation and sunset oversight committee's public comments. My family has carried the guilt of not knowing my grandmother was suffering and trusting that she would be safe in a facility. My grandmother's friends in the assisted living are vulnerable to the same lack of care since actions to correct have not been put in place. This is not uncommon in our state. Please consider expanding the commission to provide more support for residents in nursing homes. I'm grateful for the work the investigators do and hope we will continue to support them.

Another member of the public spoke after me regarding her father, a resident of a long-term care facility in Delaware. Reporting multiple complaints to the Department of Health and Social Services (DHSS), she questioned the status of complaints of neglect against assisted living facilities and investigations. She requested a follow-up answer from DHSS, but unfortunately, presenters and legislators rarely respond to public comments during the meeting. Delaware does not have transparency around the number of complaints or backlog of complaints in long-term care facilities. The most recent complaint investigation is supposed to be available on the state website, but no data on quantity is readily available. Her father's facility, Folk Manor South, closed, and the facility did not provide a discharge plan for her father. The Division of Healthcare Quality did not believe any issues occurred. Chancery Court held the facility accountable, but other state agencies did not assist. Operating in silos, departments do not work together according to her testimony. The ombudsman assigned to her father's case was removed from assignment due to her advocacy for her father. I could hear the frustration and hurt in her voice, leaving me to believe families were also operating in silos, trying to navigate the cumbersome processes for answers. Despite her pertinent questions, the meeting broke for lunch with no answers.

The next day, February 23, 2022, presented the Division of Health Care Quality (DHCQ) accomplishments. I did not join this call live or provide public comment, but all state meetings are recorded. Only 22 annual surveys for nursing homes and assisted living facilities were conducted, despite the state licensing over 80 facilities. DHCQ investigated 355 onsite complaints. Certified Nursing Assistant training was conducted by DHCQ staff for members of the National Guard to provide support to seven skilled nursing facilities short on staff. According to DHCQ, patients could not be discharged from hospitals due to a lack of staff at these facilities. The DHCQ department had a 27% vacancy rate, delaying critical work such as surveys and complaint investigations. During the open discussion by legislators, it was questioned when the most recent survey visit occurred for the Veterans Home, but the director couldn't provide an answer. Senator Sturgeon challenged who the findings of the investigation are reported to, as she was aware of cases where families do not have results. The director stated families could request the deficiency report using the Freedom of Information Act (FOIA) request, but Senator Sturgeon's constituent did not receive answers despite using the process. "Families are putting their most vulnerable members, paying a lot of money, and then when something happens and they can't get actionable information, it is concerning," stated Senator Sturgeon.

As the meeting continued, Representative Bentz challenged compliance with federal requirements for facilities certified by CMS for annual surveys. States can lose federal funding if annual surveys are not completed. While other states had lost funding, Delaware did not. Trained staff to conduct surveys was cited as a barrier to completing the work. The pay for surveyors is not competitive compared to the private market, given the extra training required, so contract surveyors were considered. Members of the National Guard who were sent to skilled nursing facilities were "unwelcomed" due to holding staff to standards they are held to, according to Representative Briggs-King. No one acknowledged the comment about being "unwelcomed," which should have been a red flag. National Guard members spent two weeks getting trained in a new healthcare setting and were able to identify gaps in care; yet, the DHCQ director claimed it takes a year of training for a nurse to perform a survey. During the public comment period, the director of the organization representing long-term care facilities, Cheryl Heiks, spoke. Workforce issues, retention, and recruitment present a challenge in long-term care. A more comprehensive plan is needed for workforce development, according to the director.

Another member of the public read the definition of the ombudsman from the state of Delaware and brought up the backlog of complaints. She described keeping up with the surveys as fiscally responsible to avoid losing federal funding. One other member of the public also spoke, expressing that she struggled with the complaint process as well. Her mother passed away in October 2021, and as of February 2022, she had not received any results. After public comment, a senator asked how many 5-star facilities were certified in the state. Unsure of the answer, the secretary of DHSS only knew of the state-run facility as 5-star certified. Additional resources were requested for the Delaware Nursing Home Residents Quality Assurance Commission, as only one person is a full-time employee; all other members volunteer. Senator Lawson described a resident of the Veterans Home who had to be admitted to the hospital with a UTI and severe dehydration. The catheter was found lying on the floor when the family came to the facility. He questioned how someone living in a long-term care facility with 24/7 staff could suffer such neglect. The secretary of DHSS claimed if the death of a resident can be traced to neglect, a facility would be classified as "immediate jeopardy," triggering additional oversight. Once we finally received the complaint investigation results, it was shown Memom died of neglect, but this classification was never given to the assisted living facility. Again, my representative failed to bring up my family's struggle with getting the investigation completed. The chairman closed the meeting, acknowledging the frequency of neglect stories brought forward, but the committee failed to make suggestions on solutions, paralyzed by the statements of workforce challenges.

Meredith- The News Journal

Emails to newspaper journalists throughout the state were not getting me anywhere, but I was convinced a front-page story would be the only way to drive legislative changes. I hadn't shared much on social media about Memom's death because I felt ashamed and angry that we did not take her out of the assisted living facility. Often, if I told someone what happened, they would quickly reply that they would have never left their loved one in the facility after the fall or being yelled at. I felt guilty and didn't want my mom to read or be subjected to judgment for our decisions. It was hard enough to question the what-ifs for every decision made without hundreds of people piling on. Another common comment was that people would sue the facility. Our experience so far was that the lawsuit wouldn't be an easy process despite the medical records, and we weren't sure it would really make a difference in preventing this from happening to someone else. After months of only a few close friends knowing the whole story, I decided to share Memom's story of neglect on Facebook. At the end of my post, I asked for anyone to help me get in contact with a newspaper reporter, as I believed neglect in long-term care facilities was rampant.

Bracing myself for people judging my family's decisions, I was hopeful at least one person would have a lead. Comments included people expressing their condolences, a few questioned why we kept Memom there, and even some other stories of neglect. One of my former high school classmates contacted me in Messenger, outraged that nurses didn't get Memom help earlier. As a nurse, she knew how painful it had to have been for Memom, even though Memom never complained. Her sister worked at The News Journal and put me in contact with an investigative journalist, Meredith Newman, in October 2021. Meredith called me, and I shared the details of Memom's story but emphasized the bigger systemic issues with long-term care facilities. From the first phone call, I knew I had finally found someone who believed in the merits of exposing the truth. We discussed ideas for information to investigate, and Meredith began researching immediately.

A lot of information about state oversight and complaints was not readily available on public websites. I only knew from speaking to other families and watching national news reports the pervasiveness of neglect in facilities. Meredith began compiling a list of information she needed and submitted Freedom of Information Act (FOIA) requests. Letters, reports, and data started to show how the state oversight processes were failing and not holding facilities accountable to standards. Some requests took months and cost hundreds of dollars to obtain, but as time went on, it was clear the wait was worth it to get the truth. I kept in contact with Meredith via texts, calls, and emails each week. Any information I received regarding Memom's investigation, I passed along to Meredith. She monitored national newspapers for stories as well, knowing Delaware had the same problems. A New York Times article, "How Nursing Homes' Worst Offenses Are Hidden From the Public," by Gebeloff, Thomas, and Silver-Greenberg, unveiled the "secretive appeals process." This article came out before we saw Memom's complaint investigation and knew about the negotiations between the state and facility on the outcomes. Several devastating neglect cases were uncovered, and investigators determined the government "didn't report the incidents to the public or factor them into its influential ratings system." Examples included "in Arizona, a nursing home resident was sexually assaulted in the dining room" and "in Texas, a woman with dementia was found in her nursing home's parking lot, lying in a pool of blood." The incidents were not rare, as the "investigation found that at least 2,700 similarly dangerous incidents were also not factored into the rating system."

Assisted living facility oversight is managed at the state level but seemed to have similar processes to the appeals process. As Meredith read more investigation reports, she confirmed the disclaimer of no legal admission to deficiencies in Memom's plan for correction seemed rare. Also, more families contacted Meredith when she shared a Facebook post looking for others impacted by neglect. Each week it became clearer a series of articles was needed to reveal the depth and complexity of failures to provide quality care. During the article development, Meredith visited me at my home to look at Memom's journals, scrapbook from her nursing career at the Hospital for the Chronically Ill, and to record answers to her questions. It surprised me with newspapers printing daily how much work goes into articles. The News Journal created a database with more than 140 reports and hundreds of pages of documents of assisted living facility inspections. From 2013 to 2022, their analysis showed the Division of Health Care Quality failed to inspect many facilities for a handful of years. In most meetings I attended, the pandemic and lockdowns were used as an excuse for any abuse or neglect, but these reports showed failure to follow standards well before it. Another interesting piece of data the investigation discovered is "in about one-third of inspections, facilities were not cited for any deficiencies." I reflected on the *New York Times* article and wondered how many deficiencies were removed in the appeals process.

Meredith attended state meetings like the Delaware Nursing Home Residents Quality Assurance Commission to learn firsthand the state process for senior care oversight. After the March 2022 meeting, I stopped attending and focused only on communicating with Meredith and my professional career. Mentally, I couldn't face any more meetings where I poured out my heart begging for changes only to hear excuses about workforce shortages, funding, and the pandemic. My scope of work in my full-time job expanded, and my health was suffering from a lack of stress management. Almost a year and a half into the journey, I knew I needed to wait for the articles before I spent time on any state meetings again.

Throughout the investigation process, Meredith asked if she could share my information with other families she connected with. Knowing my mission to advocate for change, she encountered people who wanted to honor their loved ones like I did. It was heartbreaking to listen to the stories but motivated me to keep going. On February 15, 2023, the first article in Meredith's series was published: "They thought their mother was safe in her nursing home. Then their worst fear came true." Lorece Stewart, a resident of a secured dementia unit, went missing. Her son was called to ask if she was with him, and knowing she wasn't, he went to the facility. She had fallen three stories to her death and was found outside. Meredith uncovered years of deficiencies the facility had been cited for and even that the facility was deemed to be in "immediate jeopardy" in 2011. Facilities are only in that category with patterns of quality issues causing a danger to residents. A few days after this article, Meredith published another asking the public to contact her if they had information to share.

Finally, on April 16, 2023, almost 18 months after I contacted Meredith, Memom's story was published on the front page: "She was a geriatric nurse. Why did it take Delaware so long to realize she was neglected?" The article described the events leading to Memom's death, other deficiencies found at Memom's assisted living facilities, and placed an emphasis on the decade-long struggles with the state investigating complaints. One month before Memom was hospitalized, the facility was "cited for neglect, specifically failing to pay attention to the physical needs of two residents with COVID-19." A resident with dementia was found walking the street outside the facility in July 2021. Three investigations in 2021, including Memom's, showed neglect of residents. With the struggle to get Memom's investigation completed, it made me concerned about how many other families may have given up on the process. The former Division of Health Care Quality Director, Mary Peterson, was interviewed as a part of the article. She stated the division was "underfunded during her tenure from 2013 to 2019." Even in 2013, she claimed there was a two-year backlog of complaints. This resulted in gaps in annual inspections of assisted living facilities.

Only two assisted living facilities were surveyed in 2018 and 2019 each year. A key federal report in September 2020 from the Office of the Inspector General "found that Delaware was one of 10 states that failed to meet Medicare's performance threshold for timely investigation of high-priority nursing home complaints every year from 2011 to 2018." Assisted living facilities were not included in the report, but it was clear substandard care occurred in all long-term care facilities.

Throughout the spring of 2023, Meredith published several more articles, often making the front page of the newspaper. I felt validated in knowing the systemic issues plaguing long-term care facilities, leading to so much suffering for residents, their families, and even the staff who work there. It seemed overwhelming how problems could exist for decades, and yet there were no legislative actions taken to address them. The continuous failure to adequately fund oversight or analyze root causes to prevent the same issues from occurring impacted so many people. Timing is everything, I learned, and Meredith's quest to expose the truth led to a movement for change. With the media coverage, I hoped conversations demanding improvements would start with people who could do something. In May 2023, my mom and I established a Facebook page, "Families for Community First Choice," to start sharing information about the benefits of home-based care for seniors. We used the screenshot of the newspaper story on the page to warn others of the neglect in assisted living facilities. With the information we learned, we believed the safest plan for the elderly was to avoid being institutionalized as long as possible.

Long-Term Care and Memory Care Task Force

On June 29, 2022, Concurrent Resolution 110 passed the Senate with unanimous approval, establishing the Long-Term Care and

Memory Care Task Force. Concurrent Resolutions are legislative tools to direct a group of legislators and stakeholders, including members of the public, to investigate and develop action plans for topics when it isn't clear which bills should be presented to solve an issue. Typically, task forces are created, and a series of meetings are conducted with an approved charter. The final report must be presented to the General Assembly within a certain time period. Three of the five items required to be addressed by the task force focused on staffing, one on developing additional requirements for individuals diagnosed with Alzheimer's Disease and other dementias, and the report was due by May 31, 2023. I stopped closely monitoring legislative activity in May 2022, assuming no one was listening and tired of making no progress. Senator Mantzavinos and Representative Mitchell co-led the task force. Michelle, a constituent of one of the legislators chairing the task force, inspired the need for change. Originally, there were supposed to be three members of the public as members of the task force, but somehow Michelle was the only person not involved as their paid job once the meetings started. The other seventeen voting members included legislators, long-term care facility leaders, the AARP advocacy director, the Alzheimer's Association advocacy director, and various state leaders. Some advocates I knew from other meetings decided to participate as members of the public, without a vote. They kept me informed of the meetings via text messages and emails.

Fourteen meetings were held between August 2022 and May 2023. Based on meeting minutes, long-term care industry representatives repeatedly brought up workforce shortages and staffing issues. The same conversations I listened to in meetings I attended continued to dominate these meetings. There were limited ideas to get past the staffing problems, claiming any additional requirements could put facilities in jeopardy of closing. Meetings included various presentations and prompting questions to drive discussion for developing actions. On May 3, 2023, the draft report was published. The task force generated seventeen recommendations, ranging from immediate actions to more investigative tasks. This report was reviewed and discussed in the final meeting on May 25, 2023. A few days before, I received written comments via email from Michelle, indicating how challenging it was to be a voice on a task force when she was the only member of the public. She and another advocate texted me, asking me to join the Thursday evening call. They knew I was working with Meredith on the newspaper article and had researched issues for years at this point. Work was still very busy for me, and I wasn't prepared to be let down with excuses again, but I also felt the need to support others suffering from grief. The afternoon of the meeting, I registered for public comment.

During the meeting, the seventeen recommendations were discussed, and I listened to members bring up challenges with executing them. Several of the items seemed difficult to define what would drive completion. For example, "investigate state oversight bodies' practices regarding communication with residents and family members to promote greater transparency, understanding of relevant laws and procedures, and access to relevant resources." Another item, "review oversight for assisted living facilities," seemed open-ended and unclear as to what happens after the review. While the task force developed a few specific recommendations, I had to hope the establishment of the committee on aging and eldercare would continue the conversation. Reflecting on my email to Representative Williams in February 2021, asking for the caucus on senior care, I was grateful at least the topic would be given priority in future legislative sessions. When it came to the public comment portion of the meeting, we were told only one minute would be allowed due to the number of participants. I made sure to click the "raise hand" button on the Zoom call quickly to be first for comments. With only one minute, I thanked the task force for coming up with ideas but also cautioned that the same excuses the industry brought up in these meetings were what caused me to take a break from advocacy. I didn't have time to share Memom's story other than that she died from neglect. After my time was up, a few other members of the public described their families' experiences with abuse and neglect. However, it was the first meeting I attended over the years where members of the long-term care industry outnumbered families in the general public comment portion. I was used to industry representatives having more voices on the panels or voting members but had never heard directors or management call in with feedback. The picture of care they painted implied stories like Memom's were rare and should be expected due to the age of residents. As the meeting continued, it was announced that the time changed from one minute to two minutes. I typed into the meeting chat my request for an additional minute. Once all attendees gave their comments, I was allowed another minute, which happened to be the last comment of the meeting. Furious with the gaslighting by the industry, I stated statistics from Delaware, thanks to the research done by Meredith, and said most families either didn't know how to have a voice, were ashamed to speak up, or wanted to move on with their grief. I challenged the task force to stick to the recommendations and continue the work, without knowing when I would be ready to get involved again.

Part 3

Advocating With A Team

Delaware Elder Care Advocacy Coalition

On October 30, 2023, I officially established the Delaware Elder Care Advocacy Coalition. Even though my mom and I established a Facebook group in May 2023 to focus on community-based care, we needed more families involved and a better strategy to gain traction. During the three years of my advocacy journey, I met several family members with traumatic stories of neglect and abuse of their loved ones. Some people lost their mother, and some lost their wife, but all felt determined to improve the systems for better care of seniors. Stories of hospitalizations due to severe dehydration, the use of chemical restraints such as antipsychotic medications, and injuries due to falls were common among us. The families I contacted had either been featured in newspaper stories or joined meetings such as the Delaware Nursing Home Quality Assurance Commission. A commonality between all of us was the devastation from harm to our loved ones and frustration with oversight and accountability for quality care. It had been ten days since I resigned from my full-time regulatory position, and I was in the Outer Banks relaxing with my family. A lot of factors played into my decision to quit my job, but I knew I would not fully heal from the grief of losing Memom until changes were made to care for seniors. Honoring Memom's profession as a geriatric nurse, I chose to go all in on a strategy to drive improvements by founding an official organization.

First email to group members:

Good morning,

This is Candace Esham and I have either been given your contact info by Margaret or have known you via elder care advocacy initiatives. First, I would like to say I am sorry that tragic incidents and/ or losses have brought us together. All of you are brave for honoring your loved ones by committing to do push for better care for our elders across Delaware and the US. If you would like to be removed from this group at any time please let me know. I know life priorities change for all of us and we have seasons of our life where we can dedicate more or less time.

My goal is to determine our priorities and focus our efforts to take steps to get better legislation to drive better care. There are a few upcoming events that I want to bring attention to. I know the holidays are coming up but if we would also like to meet to discuss please let me know.

Upcoming events/ initiatives:

1. *The federal government is asking for comment on Minimum Staffing Standards for Long-Term Care Facilities. Here is the link to submit a formal comment (note- there is a 5000 character limit). Submit a comment by clicking the green "Submit a formal comment" button in the top right corner. All comments must be submitted by November 6, 2023. https://www.federalregister.gov/ documents/2023/09/06/2023-18781/medicare-and-medicaid-programs-minimum-staffing-standards-for-long-term-care-facilities-and-medicaid*
2. *The Delaware Joint Finance Committee meetings are being held in*

November. There are two of importance. I will send links to the meetings as soon as they become available. This year you can attend in person, join virtually, and/or write in comments. Please remember if you choose to speak you only get 2 minutes for comment and your mic will be muted. I recommend writing your thoughts ahead of time and timing yourself.

    c. *On November 13 (10 am to 12 pm) the Department of Justice hearing for Fiscal Year 2025 will be held. This meeting will include coverage of the budget for Margaret's DNHRQAC committee. I am going to propose (again) that her department receive funding for at least one additional full time staff member to support their missions.*

    d. *On November 17 (10 am to 1 pm) the Department of Health and Social Services committee hearing for Fiscal Year 2025 will be held. I am planning on proposing a feasibility study for Community First Choice (CFC). For those of you not familiar with CFC it is a federal program that states have to apply for. Attached is a document with more details.*

3. *On Tuesday November 14, Representative Kevin Hensley hosts a Coffee Meeting from 8:30 to 9:30 at the Odessa Fire Company. Kevin is on the task force below and the Joint Finance Committee. I plan on attending and bringing up support for CFC. Kevin is my local representative and is familiar with my Memom's story (attached pdf).*

4. *On November 15 the "Enhancing Lifelong Community Supports for the Aging, Individuals with Disabilities, and Their Family Caregivers Task Force" is meeting at 1 pm (virtually). https://legis. delaware.gov/TaskForceDetail?taskForceId=452*

If I am missing any upcoming events for November, please let me know. Also, if you have any legislation you would like me to discuss at any of these events, I would be happy to. Please feel free to reach out to me directly via email or you can call my cell.

Looking forward to partnering with you all.

Thanks,

Candace

In the email, I attached the article from *The News Journal* about Memom and the backlog of complaint investigations in assisted living facilities. Initially, my focus was on improving access to community-based care to provide the best opportunity for seniors to remain at home and with loved ones. As with any successful organization, establishing a mission statement is critical to provide clarity to the goal of the group's efforts. Our first mission statement was "to provide quality support and services to elders and their families in a community-based setting so that they have the option to remain at home with loved ones." Based on the lack of problem-solving I experienced in the various state meetings, I thought tackling the complexities of long-term care facility quality would be futile. Families I knew in Delaware struggled with finding services to help their aging loved ones avoid long-term care facilities. Simple services such as assistance with meals, daycare centers for residents with dementia, and geriatric-trained specialists were lacking throughout the state. Often, families felt they had no choice but to find a facility and expressed guilt for doing so.

One by one, each of the advocates I reached out to in the email replied, excited about the forming of an official group to join efforts in making changes. A common theme between us was the lack of impact our public comments made in the various legislative meetings. Some had been speaking up for changes since 2011 and were experienced with the challenges ahead of us. The possibility of collaborating on a unified message gave hope to the group. In the emails from the members, I learned how difficult everyone's journey had been to get to this point, and it motivated me to help make a difference. I was confident the knowledge and passion from the members would give our coalition the momentum to move legislation forward. Once I received confirmation from each person on their commitment to join, I decided to expand the mission to include long-term care facility improvements. I converted the Facebook name to "Delaware Elder Care Advocacy Coalition." Based on my personal work experience in corporate structures, I began drafting a proposal for our coalition, including a mission statement, description of who we were, priorities for 2024, and key pillars. Not only would the proposal give our group focus, without overwhelming us with how broken the care system in the state is, but when we met with legislators and stakeholders, we would have legitimacy and structure. Just speaking about our personal experiences did not drive changes but researching and recommending priorities we were hopeful would. With our first official meeting scheduled for November 29th, I began to draft the proposal.

Coalition plan details

Throughout my professional career, I worked in the nuclear power industry, healthcare (major hospital system and medical device manufacturing), and the chemical manufacturing industry. All were heavily regulated; a performance improvement structure was critical to the businesses being allowed to operate and be successful. In my roles, I partnered with cross-discipline teams to develop strategies for continuous improvement each year. I formatted the proposal like how multi-million-dollar businesses operate, hoping for success. One of the coalition members created a logo with our name, the last piece we needed for legitimacy. Under the logo on the first page, I included the phrase "a proposal for legislative change to ensure our most vulnerable citizens thrive" to guide the reader on the purpose. The proposal featured our logo, a table of contents, a mission statement, a description of who we were, priorities for 2024, and key pillars. Based on the input of coalition members and the dire need for improvement, our mission statement evolved from community-focused care legislation to "promote legislation for Delaware aging residents to ensure they receive quality care and thrive." Including the focus on legislation was critical to keeping both the coalition members and the people we interacted with informed of our mission. There are so many aspects to supporting seniors, caregivers, and the systems—including workforce—that encompass the aging process that it would be easy to keep taking on initiatives outside of promoting legislation. I believed that by developing effective legislation, either by modeling off other states or even other industries, pieces of the system would have incremental improvements. We did not have the number of resources needed within our group to solve the other problems, such as the lack of caregiver support, training, and enforcing standards, and we did not want to focus only on the symptoms of the problems. As I experienced in my several years of advocacy prior, I did not want to continue with Band-Aid solutions for one-off issues and avoid the root cause.

Next, highlighting who we were, the journey that led us to form, and our beliefs behind our mission showed our solution-focused mindset and commitment to the future. The Delaware Elder Care Advocacy Coalition was formed by families who share a passion for driving legislation for aging residents to ensure quality care. Each of our families has been impacted by neglect, harm, and loss of our loved ones. We are committed to honoring our loved ones and protecting Delaware residents by promoting impactful elder care legislation. Our coalition believes in a multi-pronged approach by providing options for remain-at-home care and driving change to improve transparency, accountability, and best-in-class care through community-based elder services and improved facility-based care. We believe competition for facilities via at-home care will not only support seniors' ability to remain at home but also encourage facilities to improve their performance to ensure safe, quality care. With our public comment in state meetings limited to two minutes, it was impossible to describe the failures of care for seniors and provide ideas for change. In my experience, if I spoke about the details of Memom's neglect, either the listener didn't know what to say, attributed her death to old age, or expressed condolences without offering to work on improvements to care. We wanted to be known for partnering with stakeholders, not just trying to share our loved ones' stories.

With some members advocating over a decade and the evidence of broken processes throughout the care system, I did not want our group to feel like we needed to solve everything at once. Also, "SMART goals" were used in my professional work environments for effective goal setting in both a personal and organizational level. The acronym stands for "specific, measurable, achievable, relevant, and time-based." I chose five goals, all to be accomplished in 2024, based on experiences from other coalition members and to align with our key pillars. For each goal, I could already envision ways to accomplish it and which organizations in the state to engage with for success. Even if we did not achieve all goals, I believed showing progress on at least some would boost the confidence of coalition members and the legitimacy of our work as well as making "relevant" changes to the system. The priorities for 2024 were as follows:

1. Implement Community First Choice Option in Delaware
2. Ensure Delaware facilities comply with current laws, specifically the Centers for Medicare & Medicaid Services (CMS) requirement for annual surveys and Eagles Law
3. Implement Memory Care training as specified in Senate Bill 150 and Senate Bill 283
4. Create transparency and accountability for surveys and complaints in facilities to allow easy public access to make informed decisions on care
5. Develop regulations for assisted living facilities and memory care facilities as these are not currently covered under CMS

Details for each of the priorities were included in the report including justification for the goal with statistics and if other states already implemented the actions. The format for the proposal provided a layout for updated goals every year. We planned on establishing awareness that we were advocating for years to come and just getting started with these five goals.

Our mission statement focusing on legislation for the entire aging process, both in community and institutions, led to the development of three key pillars for the continuum of care. The goals set every year would fall into one of the pillars and ensure we were focusing on all aspects as the systems that support the aging process can be seen as an ecosystem. For example, if we only focused on community-based improvements, aging residents in long-term care facilities would not have a group advocating for legislative changes. While our plan was to at least delay the admission of loved ones to long-term care facilities as long as possible, we realized not every resident could have the support to stay at home. Both community based and institutional care needed a major overhaul, so it would've been easy to develop five goals only in one of the areas. Our key pillars are as follows:

    a. Access to quality, affordable community-based setting care

    b. Transparency and accountability for all care services

    c. Best in class care for residents at all facilities

These pillars allowed for "SMART goals" to be developed that align with words chosen intentionally to describe important qualities in each portion of the care system for residents to be able to live their best life. In the first key pillar, we chose access to related to community-based setting care. The ability to use community-based care includes not only the resources be available for the services aging residents need but also awareness they exist and the ease of families to choose this option. Memom chose to move into an assisted living facility because she spent her nursing career caring for geriatric patients, aware of the additional assistance needed as one ages and the importance of avoiding social isolation. If quality, affordable options were available to support the physical and emotional health of seniors in the community, Memom likely would not have moved into an assisted living facility. Another important key pillar applicable to both community-based and facilities is transparency and accountability. Based on our collective experience within the coalition, most families did not have an informed plan for their loved ones for aging due to lack of publicly available data and had to use what they could find to decide where to put their family member. Then, if neglect occurred, there was little recourse to drive the organization to evaluate for comprehensive corrective actions to prevent the same thing from happening to others. Perpetual harm like bed sores, wounds, and falls with injury plagued facilities. Finally, best in class encompassed cost, quality, and striving for innovative care in institutions. Throughout the years, we individually became aware of other states implementing improvement initiatives for the safety of residents and for the workforce who takes care of them. While it was obvious no state had complete model legislation, there were pieces of the process we could model in Delaware to collectively make facilities better.

Key Pillar 1: Access to quality, affordable community-based setting care

---

Mission: To provide quality services to elders and their families in a community-based setting that are essential in supporting elders' ability to remain at home and with loved ones.

My mom researched a federal program called "Community First Choice" (CFC) after reading about it in an AARP article. According to the federal government's Medicaid website, the "Community First Choice Option" allows states to provide home and community-based attendant services and supports to eligible Medicaid enrollees under their State Plan. This state plan option was established under the Affordable Care Act of 2010. Unlike other benefits in the Affordable Care Act, each state must individually apply to opt into the program. At the time of founding our coalition, only nine of all fifty states had access to this support. A website for Memory Care in Texas states, "The Community First Choice program prevents enrollees from needing to move into a nursing home through additional support services" (https://www.dementiacarecentral. com/memory-care/texas). Johns Hopkins published a study in July of 2018 with the following conclusion: "A qualitative study in the *Journal of Applied Gerontology* led by Ph.D. candidate Julia Burgdorf suggests that CFC in Maryland has been financially feasible, enhanced the personal care workforce, and supported a more equitable approach to personal care services." The program provides a six percentage point increase in federal matching payments to states for service expenditures related to the care provided. Examples of services offered in the program in every state include:

Attendant Care– When someone helps with daily activities like getting out of bed, taking a bath, getting dressed, fixing and eating meals, or using the bathroom.

Home-Delivered Meals – Nutritious meals that can be delivered fresh each day or frozen for weekends.

Personal Emergency Response System (PERS) – A call button to get help in an emergency.

Adult Day Services – A place provides supervised care and activities during the day.

Adult Day Health Services – a place that provides skilled nursing, supervised care, and activities during the day.

Facility-Based Respite Care – Short Stays in a facility so the caregiver can go on vacation.

In-Home Respite Care – Someone to stay in the loved one's home for a short time so the caregiver can get some rest.

Environmental Modifications – Changes to the home that will help seniors get around more easily and safely like grab bars or a wheelchair ramp.

The lack of availability of these services in the community in Delaware was what led families to decide to place loved ones in long-term care facilities, especially in assisted living facilities. Often, families must pay out of pocket for assisted living facility fees, averaging $7,425 per month, according to Genworth's 2023 Cost of Care Survey. For most families, the cost makes this option unachievable and forces them to make difficult financial decisions. In other states that implemented the CFC option, entrepreneurs applied for licenses to offer community-based care options, generating more availability for seniors who qualify for Medicaid and for those who wanted to pay out of pocket. Qualifying for Medicaid for long-term care programs requires the household income to be under certain limits as defined by the Federal Poverty Level, based on family size, and financial resources under a certain amount. Services in the community, if available, were a fraction of the cost of institutions, with the average hourly rate for home care in Delaware at $24 according to Genworth's 2023 Cost of Care Survey.

Community First Choice Option (CFC)

Medicare exemption overview:

Community First Choice (CFC) is a Medicaid program created by the Affordable Care Act (ACA) of 2010 to allow states to offer home- and community-based services to Medicaid beneficiaries. (The ACA added the CFC program to the Social Security Act, under Section 1915(k).) States that choose to run CFC programs will receive increased federal matching funds to provide care attendants and supports to Medicaid beneficiaries who would otherwise need to be institutionalized.

The CFC program requires states to allow Medicaid beneficiaries to direct their own care as much as possible. Under CFC, the Medicaid beneficiary should have the authority to interview care attendants, choose the best one, and fire that person if necessary.

The "Community First Choice Option" allows states to provide home and community-based attendant services and supports to eligible Medicaid enrollees under their State Plan.

This option became available on October 1, 2011, and provides a 6 percent point increase in federal matching payments to states for service expenditures related to this option. Note: Each state must individually pass legislation to request this as an exemption, and as of October 2023, elders in only nine states have access to this support, although residents of all fifty states receive all other services and benefits under the 2011 Affordable Care Act. States with the program include Arkansas, Arizona, Oregon, California, New York, Montana, Minnesota, Maryland, and Texas.

The purpose of the CFC option is to provide individuals meeting an institutional level of care the opportunity to receive necessary personal attendant services (PAS) and supports in a home and community-based setting.

The CFC option expands Medicaid opportunities for the provision of home and community-based long-term services and supports (LTSS) and is an additional tool that states can use to facilitate community integration while receiving enhanced federal matching of six (6) additional percentage points for CFC services and supports. At the time of developing the proposal, we did not know the actual cost to the state and federal government for community-based care versus institutions in Delaware. However, a report published in May 2016 by the U.S. Department of Health and Human Services claimed the CFC option as "one of many strategies states can use to shift expenditures on long-term services and supports away from institutional care and toward home and community-based services." Although this initiative would involve several stakeholders to be successful, it seemed like a win for residents, government, and local businesses.

A study "Why Do States Pursue Medicaid Home Care Opportunities? Explaining State Adoption of the Patient Protection and Affordable Care Act's Home and Community-Based Services Initiatives" conducted by Kailmon Lisa Beauregard and Edward Alan Miller, published in July 2020 in *RSF: The Russell Sage Foundation Journal of the Social Sciences*, revealed factors likely leading to decisions made regarding state participation. Factors included political, socioeconomic, and programmatic conditions. One of the most interesting political hypotheses included "states with stronger nursing home lobbies should be less likely to adopt the Affordable Care Act's Home and Community-Based Services (HCBS) provisions, all else equal." In the report, it was quoted that "92 percent of consumer advocates indicated that the LTSS system should be rebalanced away from institutions to HCBS (Grabowski et al. 2010)." While the influence of advocacy groups was not statistically significant in the study, long-term care lobbyists in Delaware drove decision-making conversations in the meetings each of my coalition members participated in over the years. Factors deemed to influence opting into the CFC program included "states with a more liberal political ideology," as association with the larger Affordable Care Act legislation may have polarized state officials. The Affordable Care Act was a highly partisan bill, and even the mention of CFC in the bill could shut down conversations. Delaware election data shows double-digit percentage wins for Democratic governor candidates since 1992, which meant the political ideology of the state should be one less barrier to CFC adoption. Until my mom researched CFC, I was not aware of the program, indicating the lack of interest. We committed to implementing CFC in Delaware as a goal despite knowing the uphill battle to get there.

During the investigation into community options, my mom also came across a document titled "Aging-in-Place Working Group Final Report," published April 29, 2022. Led by Senator Mantzavinos and Representative Griffith, a task force established in September 2021 developed actions to aid in Delawareans remaining in their homes. There were no members of the public on the task force, but the working group was comprised of fourteen representatives from state or private agencies and several legislators. Four subgroups existed to analyze specific barriers. We never knew this task force existed, and the report highlighted both the benefits of "aging-in-place" and the barriers in Delaware to improve access to services. The task force developed eleven recommendations, but it didn't seem like any had been completed.

Key Pillar 2: Transparency and Accountability for All Care Services

Transparency and accountability in following current regulations are critical to resident safety and empowering families in decision-making for the choice of facilities. The local newspaper, *The News Journal*, recently published several articles on issues with state oversight organizations enforcing regulations for nursing homes and assisted livings. Memom's story, as well as several other members within the coalition, was featured, highlighting long-standing systemic problems with significant harm to seniors.

Priorities for 2024:

1. Ensure Delaware facilities comply with current laws, specifically the Centers for Medicare & Medicaid Services (CMS) requirement for annual surveys and Eagles Law.
2. Implement Memory Care training as specified in Senate Bill 150 and Senate Bill 283.
3. Create transparency and accountability for surveys and complaints in facilities to allow easy public access to make informed decisions on care.

Ensure Delaware facilities comply with current laws, specifically the CMS requirement for annual surveys and Eagles Law.

Federal law under the Centers for Medicare & Medicaid Services (CMS) requires on-site surveys conducted on a 9 to 15-month cycle with a statewide average of 12 months. Nursing homes, which include Skilled Nursing Facilities (SNFs) and Nursing Facilities (NFs), are required to be in compliance with federal requirements to receive payment under the Medicare or Medicaid programs. Assisted living facilities, like the one Memom was a resident of, are excluded from federal regulations, and the state government is supposed to provide oversight. We believe aligning assisted living facility survey frequency is critical to ensuring the safety of residents and quality of care. The state Division of Health Care Quality received federal funding to conduct the surveys, and not following the frequency could jeopardize that funding. Surveyors utilize resident interviews, observations, and conduct record reviews to determine if facilities are in compliance with federal standards. According to the Division of Health Care Quality, in 2021, only 22 "annual" surveys were conducted out of the 81 total skilled nursing homes and assisted living facilities.

House Bill 195, introduced on June 21, 2017, and signed into law on February 14, 2018, amended the Delaware Code to change the frequency from "annual" to "regular." This change was buried amongst other amendments to the 60-page code document. Each bill contains a section called "original synopsis," which is intended to highlight the significance and intent of changes. Changing one word within the 60 pages weakened the oversight of all long-term care facilities. The bill proposed to "better protect residents of long-term care facilities by using consistent terminology, consistent practices, and updating the Code to reflect changes in related areas of the law and in how long-term care is provided to ensure that all Delawareans receiving long-term care are protected from abuse, neglect, and financial exploitation." An article,

"They trusted this assisted living to protect their mother. Then came the call on Christmas," written by Meredith Newman and published in the *Delaware News Journal* on August 8, 2023, revealed that Mary Peterson, the Division of Health Care Quality director at the time of the bill amendment, stated the change to frequency "was done because the division was 'so far behind' on surveys and did not have the resources necessary to do what was the required mission of the division." Mary claimed, "the division had to ignore annual inspections of assisted living facilities in order to get a handle on the incoming complaints and other responsibilities." The year after the law changed, 2019, the fewest number of inspections occurred, with only four conducted. Rather than allowing the division to catch up on complaints, facilities had the highest number of reported incidents of abuse and falls that same year. A backlog of complaints was not new to the division, as even in 2013 there was a complaint backlog of two years. According to a September 2020 federal report from the Office of the Inspector General, Delaware, one of 10 states, failed to meet complaint timeliness requirements in all eight years from 2011 to 2018.

With the volume of bills processed throughout the legislature, representatives and senators rely on the bill sponsor to point out substantial changes to inform their vote. Unless a legislator has expertise in the subject or constituents providing input on the bill topics, most changes are voted on based on discussions in the meetings. Based on available records of the committee and floor meetings, the inspection frequency in line 266 of the bill never rose to the discussion, and the bill became law with unanimous support from both the House and Senate. These meetings occurred before the state began recording, so details of the questions, if any, are unclear.

In a written statement provided to the journalist, the Division of Health Care Quality director stated that "during the pandemic, surveyors only visited facilities for COVID-19 infection control surveys and for issues being triaged as an immediate jeopardy issue." Routine surveys began again in 2021, though the division had a limited number of surveyors. The division's staff triaged complaints, and those identified as immediate jeopardy were the priority. Training to qualify surveyors took one year from the hire date, which only exacerbated the dire state of workforce issues. As of August 2022, the surveyor vacancy rate for the state was around fifty percent. Less than half of the employees were qualified to perform their job, with others still in training. Contract services are available to perform the work, but the $851,700 in funding for these services was denied by the governor's office for Fiscal Year 2024.

As of December 7, 2023, the following information was available on the Division of Health Care Quality website regarding surveys:

Delaware Skilled Nursing Facilities - 44 total
- 19 facilities were not in CMS compliance relative to DHCQ being in there in the last 15 months

Delaware Assisted Living Facilities – 42 total
- 15 facilities had not been visited in over 2 years
- 5 have never been visited since opening
- 2 haven't been visited since 2017
- 1 hasn't been visited since 2011

Eagles Law

In 2000, state legislation following nursing home reform was created to establish staffing ratios. Delaware legislature has suspended the nursing home staffing ratio requirement, also known as Eagles Law, until

July 1, 2024. This was suspended during the pandemic due to the State of Emergency, however the State of Emergency ended in early 2023. An amendment wasn't made to the code, but language was included in the 329-page Fiscal Year 2024 Appropriations Act to waive the requirement. On 195-page 179 section 187 states, *"Long-term care facilities must continue to provide 3.28 hours of direct care per resident 4 per day. However, the staffing ratios required in 16 Del. C. 1162 are hereby suspended until July 1, 2024."* Per code: "If a nursing facility cannot meet the shift ratios due to building configuration or any other special circumstances, they may apply for a special waiver through the Division, subject to final approval by the Delaware Nursing Home Residents Quality Assurance Commission (DNHRQAC)." A subcommittee was created to review the waivers, but none had been provided as of October 2023. Unlike other changes to Delaware code for long-term care facilities, a committee hearing was not held to engage comments from key stakeholders. Also, Eagles Law only applies to skilled nursing facilities, allowing assisted living facilities to operate with no regulations on staffing ratios.

Implement Memory Care training as specified in Senate Bill 283 and Senate Bill 150

Two bills, one signed by the Governor in 2022 and one introduced in June 2023, were created to specify training for dementia care services. Senate Bill 283, sponsored by Senator Mantzavinos, intended to modify continuing education requirements for medical professionals licensed by the Board of Medical Licensure and the Board of Nursing. It added a requirement for practitioners licensed by these Boards who treat adults with dementia to complete one hour of continuing education in each reporting period on the topic of diagnosis, treatment, and care of patients with Alzheimer's disease or other dementias. This bill was modeled on legislation in Massachusetts and was written to cover medical professionals outside of long-term care facilities who provide care for dementia residents.

In the first of four meetings, a geriatric psychologist testified in support of the bill, stating Delaware is home to about 190,000 residents aged 65 and older, comprising 19.5% of the state population. Delaware currently has 18 geriatricians, and only five other states have fewer specialists per resident. This leaves most senior residents relying on primary care physicians, which means dementia may go undiagnosed without proper training. Also in this meeting, the senior director of advocacy for the Alzheimer's Association and two family advocates explained the benefits of this bill in relation to their personal journeys. The executive director of the Delaware Nurses Association was the first to speak against the bill, claiming no consensus on benefits for training. He was followed by the President of the Medical Society of Delaware, who opposed it as well, claiming specialists already receive training and those not specializing in it do not. The geriatric psychologist who spoke at the beginning already provided data that the number of specialists in Delaware would not be able to keep up with the number of patients in the state. A member of the Delaware Healthcare Association, which represents Delaware hospitals, expressed concerns about the lack of flexibility for continuing education if it is legislated. Mary Peterson, the former Division of Healthcare Quality director, spoke in support of the bill, restating the lack of specialists available. Finally, the director for the Delaware Division of Professional Regulation claimed the department would have no way to enforce the requirement as they do not keep track of patient records. With the bill focusing on practitioners who treat adults, there would be no ability to audit.

During the Senate meeting on June 9, 2022, ten senators expressed interest in being co-sponsors in support of the bill. The only challenging comments were from Senator Sturgeon, who received feedback from a constituent with experience in the medical field who questioned the bill, as they were aware of several illnesses that lead to death where one hour of training isn't required. As in the previous hearing committee, it seemed as if medical providers were the main opposition to the bill. Despite the expert opinion of a geriatric psychologist, medical practitioners with general experience did not feel the education requirement would be enforceable or necessary for the care of adult patients. Senator Sturgeon abstained from voting, and all other present senators voted yes.

The House Committee, held on June 16, 2022, ironically discussed the Delaware Nursing Home Residents Quality Assurance Commission as a topic for first discussion. House Bill 438 expanded the requirements for the commission's annual report with more specific criteria. This report included descriptions of advocacy efforts and goals for the upcoming year, a rubric, criteria, findings, and recommendations from each facility visit, as well as aggregate data with analysis and monitoring of trends in the quality of care and quality of life of nursing home residents. The bill was approved to move through committee, other required meetings, and was signed by the Governor. Even though this was effective October 26, 2022, the annual report for 2023 was not available on the commission's website as of June 9, 2024. Senate Bill 283 was the last item on the agenda and was discussed by Senator Mitchell. He started out explaining that he found two or three things to do, but as a result, half a dozen other things needed to be addressed. Having said that, he believed the bill was critical for medical providers to strengthen their knowledge of dementia. Senator Mitchell also heard from providers who felt the training was unnecessary, but he had personal experience and feedback from families on the need for training. The chair of the committee was a current caregiver for a loved one and believed the training would benefit families.

Katie Macklin, the senior director of advocacy for the Alzheimer's Association, spoke to rebut the three arguments from opponents to the bill. First, providers challenged why dementia was chosen specifically. Only 45% of people living with dementia in Delaware received a diagnosis, leading to increased doctor and hospital visits due to a lack of understanding of the care plan. Second, dementia patients go see specialists, so why have general practitioners trained? As mentioned in the first committee meeting, Delaware is among the states with the fewest geriatric and neurology specialists in the entire country. Finally, claims of increasing continuing education requirements were swirling. The bill did not add to the total quantity but requires one of the hours to be dedicated to dementia training. A member of the public testified that her mother was not diagnosed properly despite going to primary care doctors. She participated in a five-year steering committee for Alzheimer's and learned about the lack of education doctors receive, leading to physicians being uncomfortable diagnosing a disease they knew little about. Watching members of her own church struggle with their family's journey led her to advocate for better training. They expressed wanting to have a diagnosis earlier to allow for a better ability to plan financially and for healthcare. Struggling to speak through sobbing, another person described her mother receiving a misdiagnosis of attention deficit disorder by a primary care physician, then a neurologist inaccurately diagnosing her mother with Lewy body dementia, a specific type of dementia, causing her to be turned away from every care facility. A fire in the home due to a bagel forced into a toaster and caregiver break-ins only added to the stress of the disease. Her mother eventually received an accurate diagnosis of Alzheimer's, but when her mom had to go to the hospital, the unit dedicated to taking care of patients with dementia would be full. In the other units, she found her mother physically restrained and experienced issues with caregivers not knowing how to work with her mother. Her hardest interactions were with medical providers not trained on the disease. None of the opponents to the bill attended the meeting, and the bill passed through the committee.

On June 30, 2022, the bill finally made it to the House floor agenda. As it was the last day of the legislative session, the bill had to either be approved, or the process would start over in January 2023. Meetings continued until 2 in the morning to push through as many bills as possible. The bill was described to include medical professionals licensed by the Board of Medical Professionals, but the actual language within the bill only included those licensed by the Board of Nursing. The intent of bills is not always described in the final bill language appropriately. Nurses and doctors were both intended to be the targets receiving the training, as nurses are not licensed to perform diagnosis. Minimal discussion occurred in the House floor meeting, with one representative acknowledging how many families would benefit from the training requirements. With an amendment proposed, the bill went back to the Senate floor at 10 p.m. with only a few hours left to pass. All 21 senators voted yes to the bill, and it was signed by the Governor into law on September 8, 2022.

At the time of writing the proposal, I relied on input from my coalition members on priorities. Obviously, training improvements were needed based on their personal stories, but I incorrectly assumed, based on the rigorous process of developing a law, that the intended changes would be made. My family did not have experience with a loved one who had dementia, but several times, Memom was misdiagnosed with dementia. This led to different care decisions in the hospital, including tying her down by her hands and feet without us knowing. In June 2024, I watched the recordings of the meetings and investigated the code changes made because of this law. Even though the "original synopsis" and verbal description of the bill in meetings included doctors and the Board of Medical Licensure and Discipline, the text of the bill only included changes to continuing education in the Board of Nursing. These requirements were limited to "nurses who work in adult gerontology must complete at least one hour in the diagnosis, treatment, and care of patients with Alzheimer's disease or other dementias." Despite the testimony from families regarding issues in general hospital units and primary care practices, the scope focused on adult gerontology. Within the final bill itself, there was conflicting language, with one section stating those who work in "adult or gerontology" and another more specifically stating "all nursing professionals who work in adult gerontology." This would exclude nursing professionals who worked in the emergency department, primary care, surgical units, or other common settings where a patient with dementia may need to go. Unfortunately, the intent of the continuing education to improve the diagnosis of dementia and interactions with patients in a non-specialist setting would not be accomplished with the new law.

Senate Bill 150 focused on staffing and training in long-term care facilities specifically. Despite the growing number of dementia care providers in the state, the Delaware Code covering long-term care facilities and services does not include memory care or dementia-care services. Excluding these critical services from the regulation provides no requirements for facilities that care for patients with dementia, despite the facilities charging up to $16,000 per month out of pocket. Senate Bill 150 was discussed in the Senate Health & Social Services Committee on June 14, 2023, sponsored by Senator Mantzavinos. The long-term care task force developed the recommendation for the bill. This Act defines dementia care services and activity services, and it requires that all long-term care facilities that offer dementia care services have "sufficient" staff to meet the needs of each resident, including a "sufficient" number of dedicated activity staff. This Act also requires that the staff who work with residents receiving dementia care services complete twelve hours of dementia care training and identifies certain requirements for such training. During the committee hearing, legislators had several questions. The definition of "sufficient" staff and how to enforce it was challenged. The deputy secretary of the Division of Health & Social Services stated "annual" surveys would determine if facilities complied with the staffing needs. No one corrected the deputy secretary on the misstatement of frequency. Also, a senator stated the legislation seemed "fuzzy," given the harsh penalty with the threat of closure. The secretary of the Division of Health & Social Services was in attendance as well and explained that the word "sufficient" was chosen based on federal language purposely vague to allow individual plans of care. Each resident had unique needs, and the number of staff for direct care varied accordingly.

Staffing standards drove the conversation at the hearing even though training requirements were an important aspect of the bill. Almost thirty minutes of senator discussion passed before moving to public comment. One of the facility directors stated, "We are an industry in crisis," claiming extensive training requirements will remove staff from providing resident care. The staffing "crisis," lack of funding, and an emphasis on direct care continued as a theme throughout industry member comments. Seven representatives from the long-term care industry testified in person against the timing of the bill. The government affairs director for the Alzheimer's Association claimed the bill "makes the lives of those living with the disease easier" and ensures staff at facilities can safely interact, potentially leading to the life or death of a resident. One of my coalition members was the only family advocate who spoke during public comment, addressing the importance of protecting these vulnerable residents. Ultimately, the six senators supported moving the bill out of committee "on its merits," and one senator asked for his name to be removed from the sponsorship due to the volume of comments. Senator Mantzavinos promised to work with stakeholders on an amendment to incorporate feedback. At the time of the proposal development, it was unclear when the bill would be revisited, but we included this in the coalition priorities.

Families believed medical providers would understand the best practices to diagnose and care for patients with dementia, but their journey with their loved ones proved this theory wrong. Caregivers became the experts through living with their loved ones and were continuously let down by the medical system. We strongly recommended involving caregivers and family members of those with dementia in the development of the training. They have first-hand experience of the skills needed to provide quality, safe, respectful care to those with dementia. There are several support groups that would be willing to provide time and knowledge for the development of valuable training programs. Lack of appropriate training can have severe consequences for the residents with dementia and the staff who are providing care for them.

Create transparency and accountability for surveys
and complaints in facilities to allow easy public
access to make informed decisions on care

Families do not have easy access to the survey and complaint data to help them in their decision-making. Individuals can request results via the Freedom of Information Act (FOIA), but there are no guarantees the results will be released, and requests can cost money. For example, family members who are not the power of attorney do not have rights to the information. While this is intended to protect the residents of facilities, sometimes the power of attorney does not want to pursue answers to complaints, leaving other family members wondering what led to the harm. I experienced this when trying to find the investigation of the fall Memom had in August 2020. Without my uncle's agreement to get the document, I never knew if the investigation was even completed. In addition, requesting results one at a time can be time-consuming and does not allow a full picture of the quality of care at these facilities. Access to information on the safety and quality of facilities is critical for families to make informed decisions on where to have their loved one live, as well as to hold facilities accountable for making improvements.

When we were deciding as a family the best assisted living facility for Memom, my mom looked up available information on complaints and violations for facilities in the Dover area. Memom had been a member of Christ Episcopal Church in Dover for decades and wanted to be able to keep attending services there. I was christened there, and several family members, including my parents, got married there. The facility Memom and the family chose was based on no complaints being available. Other facilities in the area had dozens of serious complaints, and we assumed the lack of complaints listed meant exceptional care. Years later, we discovered that lots of factors could lead to a lack of complaints, including outdated data, families not knowing how to file complaints, or even families fearing retaliation if complaints were filed.

Key Pillar 3: Best in class care for residents at all facilities

---

Priority for 2024: Develop regulations for Assisted Living facilities and memory care facilities as these are not currently covered under Centers for Medicare & Medicaid Services (CMS).

Federal government regulations under CMS do not cover assisted living facilities. Oversight and accountability are needed for these facilities to ensure adequate care is provided. Common arguments for the need for more regulations included assisted living facilities not being medical facilities, residents moving in for the social environment, and workforce shortage issues. Other states have implemented laws for assisted living facilities, and we encouraged these best practices in our proposal. Each of our members was told for years about the difficulty or lack of need to change assisted living facility regulations. However, in our research, states all over the country were committed to enforcing higher standards of care. Dementia and memory care aren't even defined in Delaware code, meaning there are no regulations for these services. It became clear in our search for best practices how much improvement was needed in Delaware regulations on assisted living facilities.

Arkansas

100 (arkansas.gov)

Regulations in the state of Arkansas include specific requirements for staffing plans to meet the needs of residents, training topics such as dementia and cognitive impairment, incident reporting, and quarterly quality assurance reviews. All staff members and consultants shall have dementia training, unlike in Delaware, where current regulations only specify requirements for certified nursing assistants. Thirty hours of training requirements are listed, with ongoing in-service training of at least two hours every quarter. The 114-page document provides extensive details to guide facilities to quality care.

Colorado

Bill Text: CO SB079 | 2022 | Regular Session | Enrolled | LegiScan

Senate Bill 79 was passed on May 31, 2022, for dementia training for direct-care staff of specified facilities that provide services to clients living with dementia. In the bill, it is stated that dementia training can "more adequately prepare direct-care staff for the responsibilities of these jobs, potentially reducing stress, staff burnout, and turnover." At least four hours of initial dementia training is required, and at least two hours of continuing education on dementia topics for all direct-care staff members every two years. Specific topics listed are dementia diseases and related disabilities, person-centered care, care planning, and dementia-related behaviors and communication. Both nursing homes and assisted living facilities licensed by the state of Colorado were within the scope of the training requirements.

North Carolina

reports.oah.state.nc.us/ncac/title 10a - health and human services/ chapter 13 - nc medical care commission/subchapter f/subchapter f rules.html

Both staffing ratios and training requirements are specified in assisted living facility regulations. For units providing memory care, at least one staff member is required for every eight residents on the first and second shifts. One staff member for every ten residents is mandated on the third shift. Training for staff working in these units includes six hours of orientation within the first week of employment, twenty hours of dementia-specific training within six months of employment, and twelve hours of continuing training annually.

Oregon

HB3359 (oregonlegislature.gov)

In 2017, Oregon revised regulations for long-term care facilities, including assisted living facilities. An acuity-based staffing tool was developed to "determine whether they have a sufficient number of qualified awake caregivers to meet the 24-hour scheduled and unscheduled needs of each resident." Also, all direct care staff, prior to providing direct care to residents of the facility, must complete training in dementia care. This includes education on the dementia disease process, techniques for understanding and managing behavioral symptoms, strategies for addressing social needs, and ways to ensure the safety of residents. A special memory care endorsement is required for facilities that advertise or market providing dementia care.

Future priorities: Technology

We included a section on technology in the proposal to highlight best practices we found throughout the country. One of my coalition members utilized his personal and professional experience to research options. With facility directors constantly using workforce shortages as a barrier to providing better care, we researched technological advancements to aid staff and residents.

Promoting Effective Family Communication and
Technological Advancements in Care Facilities
Harnessing Technology for Easy and Effective Communication
Incorporating user-friendly technologies, such as video phones, to facilitate seamless communication between caregivers and the families of residents is paramount. These technologies must be designed with simplicity in mind, catering to the needs of the elderly, including those suffering from dementia or cognitive decline. By enhancing communication, we can significantly boost the mental well-being of both the residents and their caregivers while also fortifying facilities to handle potential future crises, such as pandemics.

In Delaware, not all facilities allow cameras in resident rooms.

Several states, including Illinois, Kansas, Minnesota, New Mexico, Oklahoma, Texas, Washington, and Louisiana, allow for cameras in nursing homes. <u>Article for State of Louisiana bill</u> Beebe Healthcare in Sussex County, Delaware uses audio/ video patient monitoring systems and has become the top 10% in the nation for reducing falls. However, these systems also have other uses. Preventing resident on resident attacks, helping the visually impaired receive assistance etc. <u>Beebe Healthcare article</u>.

Embracing Technological Advancements

It's imperative for health inspectors to enforce the utilization of up-to-date technology within care facilities. Modern technology not only elevates the quality of care but also optimizes staff efficiency, ensuring that residents receive the best possible support. <u>Automation article</u>

Revamping Nurse Call Bell Systems

Nurse call bell systems should be integrated with mobile devices, ensuring all nursing staff are equipped for communication. When a resident activates the call button, the message is instantly relayed to the nurse, wherever they are in the facility. These systems must also feature comprehensive reporting capabilities for assessing residents' needs and response times. Two-way communication between residents and nurses is essential to discern the nature of assistance required, whether it's a simple drink of water or a more critical medical issue. Furthermore, two-way communication with other nurses is vital, enabling collaboration without leaving the patient's side. These devices should be capable of sending code alerts to all nurses and doctors, such as in the case of a resident falling, and maintain the ability to signal a facility lockdown during emergencies like active shooter incidents.

Leveraging Cutting-Edge Technology for Enhanced Care

Embracing Smart Beds

Incorporating smart beds with integrated sensors is a game changer in healthcare. These innovative beds can relay critical patient data, such as heart rate and respiration, directly to the nursing staff. Moreover, they aid in patient repositioning, reducing the risk of painful bedsores. Some models even feature mattresses that automatically adjust to relieve pressure areas, ensuring patient comfort and well-being.

Seizing the Potential of Tablets

Harnessing the power of tablets in healthcare is a remarkable advancement. Tablets empower nursing staff to efficiently enter patient information right from the resident's room. This data is seamlessly integrated into the system as soon as it's submitted via the tablet, eliminating the need for time-consuming rounds, handwritten notes, and redundant data entry into a computer. This technology streamlines the workflow, allowing healthcare providers to focus on what matters most: caring for the residents.

Establishment of Specialized Teams and Enhanced Family Involvement

Formation of Specialized Teams

Care facilities should establish dedicated teams for safe and proper patient transfers, whether from a bed to a wheelchair or for bathing, ensuring residents' well-being.

Facilitate Family Involvement

In addition to resident councils, it's essential for facilities to create family councils to encourage families to contribute their insights for facility and patient care improvements. These channels of communication will empower nursing home administrations to make informed enhancements.

Proactive Patient Monitoring and Enhanced Security Measures

Proactive Patient Monitoring: A Vital Lifeline

Implementing proactive patient monitoring technology is a cornerstone of advanced healthcare. These systems not only enhance safety but also provide essential support for patients with unique needs. In addition to the primary benefits of preventing falls and intervening before injuries occur, these systems play a crucial role in supporting patients with disabilities. For instance, they serve as a lifeline for blind patients who may have difficulty locating the nurse call bell system, ensuring their urgent requests for assistance are promptly addressed.

Furthermore, proactive monitoring extends to scenarios where patients may face immediate health risks, such as choking. By swiftly detecting such situations, these systems provide the staff with the crucial time needed to intervene and avert potential emergencies. This technology acts as an ever-vigilant guardian, significantly enhancing patient well-being and safety in care facilities.

Enhancing Patient Security

Facilities should invest in security systems that promptly alert authorities to unauthorized door openings, specifying which door has been breached.

Support for Dementia Patients

Dementia patients require wander guard technology equipped with building GPS locations. This enables staff to quickly locate and reorient residents who may have wandered off.

In summary, these recommendations collectively contribute to the enhancement of patient care quality, the optimization of operational efficiency, and the alleviation of burdens on the staff. By embracing these technological advancements, care facilities can elevate the overall quality of care provided to their residents while streamlining their internal processes for a more effective and responsive healthcare environment. Moreover, these systems not only enhance patient safety but also empower nursing staff to deliver more personalized, one-on-one care to their loved ones, fostering a nurturing and compassionate environment in which residents thrive.

Addendum

At the end of the proposal, we included an addendum with more details on each state currently using the Community First Choice (CFC) program for community-based services. Contact links and synopses of the program coverage, as well as the benefits to residents and state budgets, were highlighted in all participating states (Arkansas, Arizona, California, Connecticut, Maryland, Minnesota, Oregon, Montana, and Texas). Colorado is currently working to implement CFC by July 1, 2025. All states provided similar services to give residents the freedom to direct their own care and allow them to remain safely in their own homes.

Specifically, Oregon claimed:

"With CFC, more residents of Oregon are able to receive long-term home and community benefits from Medicaid. This is a win-win. Seniors are able to receive the care they need to continue to live at home or in the home of a family member rather than be placed in an institution, and the state saves money by avoiding the need to pay for more costly, nursing home care. That being said, eligible applicants may also choose to receive services outside of their homes, such as in an adult foster care home, adult group home, in assisted living, or a memory care home for persons with Alzheimer's."

The addendum also included two studies: the Johns Hopkins study

(Davis, Willink, Stockwell, Whiton, Burgdorf, and Woodcock, 2018), which found improved quality of care and fiscal responsibility, and another study conducted by Elizabeth Dickey, J.D., of the University of Virginia School of Law, "Understanding Medicaid's Community First Choice Program."

Another task force

Since I committed to attending all state meetings where I could introduce the coalition's purpose, I made a list of any relevant task forces to join. The "Enhancing Lifelong Community Supports for the Aging, Individuals with Disabilities, and Their Family Caregivers Task Force" was established in June 2023. I reviewed the task force goals and decided the task force should be willing to discuss the Community First Choice option to support home-based care. The third meeting, held on November 15, 2023, was only 25 minutes from my house at a local library. My local senator co-chaired the committee, and I was hopeful she would meet with me to discuss the coalition's proposal. Despite advocating for over three years, it was the first meeting dedicated to problem-solving that I was able to attend in person. Most of the discussion focused on caregivers of adult children with disabilities. The task force title included "aging," but it seemed the scope of the charter involved two very different populations. I was the only person who spoke up about seniors and gave my two-minute comments after listening for almost two hours.

I described our coalition group of volunteers and current support of ten families. I stated we were looking to expand and make improvements to facility and institutional care through a community-based, community-first option and choice. In my comments, I had to quickly explain my personal experience with Memom's neglect in an assisted living facility and her tragic death. I highlighted some details of the Community First Choice Option offered through Medicaid, created by the Affordable Care Act of 2010. My goal was to emphasize Delaware is not utilizing this program and that it could help Delawareans remain at home instead of in costly facilities. The level of care will never be the same as if it was at the individual's home versus an institution.

After the meeting, I introduced myself to a few people in the room. The policy director for the Department of Health & Social Services, Jules, was sitting a few chairs down from me. She gave me her business card and offered to connect to learn more about the coalition. Even though I didn't get any offers to meet with legislators, including my senator, I knew Jules would be a key stakeholder who understood the process to make changes. Brandon, aide to Senator Mantzavinos, attended and introduced himself. He facilitated the long-term care task force meetings and was excited a group of advocates had formed. Rita Landgraf, a leader in the American Association of Retired Persons (AARP) Delaware, also mentioned discussing our mission and providing some history on why the Community First Choice option was never implemented. I attended another task force meeting in December 2023, attempting again to examine the CFC waiver as an option, but no one added it as an action item. It seemed like meeting Jules and Brandon would be the most productive aspect of attending these meetings, and I wasn't able to change the conversation to include seniors. I decided not to attend any more of these meetings and look for other avenues to have my voice heard.

First Legislator meeting as a coalition

The final report for the Long-Term Care and Memory Care Task Force included one additional recommendation: "establish a stakeholder group to meet regularly to provide a forum for continued public engagement on issues related to long-term care." On November 7, 2023, several family members involved in advocacy, including several in my coalition, were invited to a Zoom meeting with Senator Mantzavinos, Representative Johnson, and Brandon, aide to the Senator. Held on December 5, 2023, attendees were frustrated with the number of open actions from the task force and were losing hope that things would change. Some family members had begun advocating for changes as long as fifteen years prior, with no new legislation as a result of their work. Industry lobbyists were a part of the task force and emphasized that unless more money and more people were dedicated to their organizations, changes could not occur. Senator Mantzavinos and Representative Johnson had never spoken with me directly before, but I was hopeful they were genuine since they ensured only families were invited to the meeting. I seized the opportunity with this meeting to formally introduce the name and mission statement of our coalition. Since many of my members were on the call, Senator Mantzavinos asked if I was willing to be the point of contact for families. I couldn't believe that after years of speaking up, a legislator finally recognized the value of advocates' input. He mentioned the Department of Health & Social Services project to redo their website, which would help with a coalition goal for transparency. Families, including mine, attempted to research facility metrics before choosing where to put their loved ones. Easy website navigation is key to providing the public with information on quality. We were asked to put together a proposal for website changes, and I committed to sending it by Friday, December 8, 2023. I could tell not everyone on the call felt as confident as I did in the opportunity to partner with legislators. Most had meeting fatigue from attending fourteen meetings with no updates since May 2023. However, I believed it was perfect timing to share our proposal and support as a unified voice for families. In the email to Senator

Mantzavinos and Brandon, I included our coalition's proposal and the website changes in two separate documents. With our logo as the first page, these files looked official and were taken seriously.

Proposal for DHSS Website changes for metrics
Prepared on December 8, 2023

Scope: The proposal is split into metrics currently required to be reported to Division of Health Care Quality (DHCQ), metrics tracked by facilities but not required to be reported, and metrics we would like to see required (regulation changes needed). The metrics currently required to be reported do not include Assisted Living facilities and memory care facilities. Legislation must be proposed and implemented to require these facilities to report the same as nursing home facilities and skilled nursing home facilities. We believe transparency and accountability for these metrics will provide residents and families the resources to make informed decisions on care. These metrics are not currently readily available to the public.

To enhance transparency, we requested the Division of Health Care Quality post on a website crucial data to allow families to make informed decisions on care. We divided the metrics currently required to be reported to Division of Health Care Quality (DHCQ), metrics tracked by facilities but not required to be reported, and metrics we would like to see required (regulation changes needed). The metrics currently required to be reported do not include Assisted Living facilities and memory care facilities. Legislation must be proposed and implemented to require these facilities to report the same as nursing home facilities and skilled nursing home facilities.

Metrics required to be reported to Division of Health Care Quality (DHCQ):

1. DHCQ survey results (annual and complaints)
2. Reportable incidents (number, investigation results, and average time to complete investigation):

    a. Abuse as defined in 16 Delaware Code, §1131.
- Physical abuse with injury if resident to resident and physical abuse with or without injury if staff to resident or any other person to resident.
- Any sexual act between staff and a resident and any non-consensual sexual act between residents or between a resident and any other person such as a visitor.
- Emotional abuse whether staff to resident, resident to resident or any other person to resident.

    b. Neglect, mistreatment or financial exploitation as defined in 16 Delaware Code, §1131.

    c. Resident elopement under the following circumstances:
- A resident's whereabouts on or off the premises are unknown to staff and the resident suffers harm.
- A cognitively impaired resident's whereabouts are unknown to staff and the resident leaves the facility premises.
- A resident cannot be found inside or outside a facility and the police are summoned.

    d. Significant injuries.
- Injury from an incident of unknown source in which the initial investigation or evaluation supports the conclusion that the injury is suspicious. Circumstances which may cause an injury to be suspicious are: the extent of the

injury, the location of the injury (e.g., the injury is located in an area not generally vulnerable to trauma), the number of injuries observed at one particular point in time, or the incidence of injuries over time.

- Injury which results in transfer to an acute care facility for treatment or evaluation or which requires periodic neurological reassessment of the resident's clinical status by professional staff for up to 24 hours.
- Areas of contusions or bruises caused by staff to a dependent resident during ambulation, transport, transfer or bathing.
- Significant error or omission in medication/treatment, including drug diversion, which causes the resident discomfort, jeopardizes the resident's health and safety or requires periodic monitoring for up to 48 hours.
- A burn greater than first degree.
- Any serious unusual and/or life-threatening injury.

   e. Entrapment which causes the resident injury or immobility of body or limb or which requires assistance from another person for the resident to secure release.

3. Hours Per Resident Day (HPRD)
4. Staff to patient ratio
5. Licensed/Certified per shift (nurses and Certified Nursing Assistants)
6. Percent of staff CPR/AED certified
7. Assaults (physical/sexual, patient to patient and/or staff to patient)

Metrics tracked by facilities but not required to be reported to DHCQ:

1. Incident reports retained in facility files only (number, report details, and length of time to do investigation):

   a. Falls without injury and falls with minor injuries that do not require transfer to an acute care facility or neurological reassessment of the resident.

   b. Errors or omissions in treatment or medication.

   c. Injuries of unknown source.

   d. Lost items which are not subject to financial exploitation.

   e. Skin tears.

   f. Bruises of unknown origin.

2. Complaints (number and severity)

   a. Percentage of complaints investigated

   b. Average time from date complaint submitted to investigation completion

3. Number of Employed Registered Nurses (RNs)

4. Number of Employed Licensed Practical Nurses (LPNs)

5. Number of Employed Certified Nursing Assistants (CNAs)

6. Number of Contracted RNs

7. Number of Contracted LPNs

8. Number of Contracted CNAs

Metrics not currently required to be tracked:

1. Percent of staff who have completed the required training as specified in SB 283

2. Reporting of Nurse Call Bell Response times

After receiving the information, Brandon provided me with a date and time to meet with Senator Mantzavinos. I traveled to Legislative Hall in Dover to discuss my coalition's proposal and bills for the 2024 legislative session. For the first time in over three years, I felt confident that changes would be made and advocates' voices would be heard. I committed to fully supporting negotiations and providing testimony through June 2024.

Representative Williams December and January

It had been over two years since I last spoke to Representative Williams, but her sympathy in 2021, when I spoke about Memom in the Joint Finance Committee hearing, meant a lot to me. In December, I emailed her a copy of our coalition proposal and asked for a meeting. She responded quickly, as always, and mentioned she had received extra responsibilities as co-chair of the Joint Finance Committee. Her aide met with me virtually in early January and listened to me explain the coalition's goals. Also, I had been researching where state and federal taxpayer money was being spent to try to understand how much it cost to have a senior in a long-term care facility versus providing financial assistance with community-based care. I read that other states implemented policy changes to help seniors remain at home longer, but I wanted specific data on Delaware. The documents I found on the state website regarding funding were unclear, and I hoped Representative Williams could help since she was a member of the JFC. I sent the following email on January 30, 2024:

Hi Representative Williams and Justin,

Hope you are both doing well. I had a few questions regarding the FY24 budget and hoping you can answer them or help point me in the right direction.

1. *In HB 195, there was a line item of $5 million for long-term care skilled nursing facilities, leveraging another $7.5 million in federal funds. Do you know if that money has been paid yet? What is the purpose of that money? I can't find documentation to specify what it is for. (https://housedems.delaware.gov/2023/06/22/house-passes-5-6-billion-operating-budget-for-fiscal-2024/)*

2. *For FY24, how much Medicaid money from the state was allocated for long term care facilities? Same question for federal Medicaid money.*

3. *For FY24, how much Medicaid money from the state is dedicated to community-based care for the aging (via MCO plan)? Same question for federal Medicaid money.*

If you don't know, can you help point me to who can? I have been trying to sift through documents but no luck.

Thanks,

Candace Esham

A week later I received a response which caused me to have even more questions. According to a letter written on December 21, 2023 by the Acting Director, Division of Managed Care Policy Center for Medicaid and Children's Health Insurance Program (CHIP) Services, the additional funding was for a "uniform increase established by the state for nursing facility services." The total dollar amount approved for the separate payment is actually $25,464,731, not the $12.5 million approved by the Joint Finance Committee. I assumed based on the newspaper publication this money would be used for all long-term care facilities but upon reading the form, I discovered only skilled nursing facilities would receive money. It was unclear as to how the money more than doubled after the budget review. The estimated federal share of this state directed payment was $15,464,731 and estimated non-federal share of this state directed payment was $10,000,000. Attached to the letter was a form called "Section 438.6(c) Preprint" which provided a standard federal template for how the funds were to be managed. On page eight of the form, the reason for this increase is "due to the lingering effects of the COVID-19 pandemic and impact on workforce retention and associated strain on Delaware's nursing facilities." The form included a table to put quality strategy goals and objectives in the payment arrangement, but no objectives were required for workforce retention (such as retention rate of staff). The only objectives were to "maintain access and availability for nursing facility members/ residents" and "increase member ability of getting needed care and increase members' rating of health plan." Even the example in the template included measurable objectives; "increase the number of managed care patients receiving follow-up behavioral health counseling by 15%." However, the state did not place any quantifiable metrics in that section. Therefore, any improvement to increase would be considered satisfactory.

The money had not been paid yet, but as of December 2023, this was approved as a state-directed payment. The Division of Medicaid and Medical Assistance (DMMA) planned to pay out 75% of the funds within the first quarter of the calendar year 2024. There was no requirement to prove the funds would be used for workforce retention issues, and it is unclear how "associated strain" from the pandemic can be quantified. Based on my other questions regarding how much Medicaid money was allocated for long-term care facilities versus community-based care, I learned I did not phrase them properly to get answers. Instead of gaining information about how much of the state budget was used for these programs, I was given a link to the methodology for federal funding. Even though I didn't know the breakdown of the budget, learning about the significant increase in funding for long-term care skilled nursing facilities and the lack of specificity regarding where the money could be used shed light on the lack of oversight and transparency.

January 2024

The second session of the 152nd General Assembly for the State of Delaware convened on Tuesday, January 9, 2024. Since I committed to supporting several bills during this session, I had to dive into the details of the approval process. One of my coalition members had been advocating for and monitoring bills for years, so he mentored me as well as developed a tracking tool. Each general assembly time period consists of two sessions, January to June, in consecutive years. Legislators had from January 9 to June 30 to sponsor bills through the legislative process. Some bills proposed in the first session, which occurred from January to June 2023, did not fully complete the process due to a lack of support. Any legislation from the first session could be amended, continue the process through committees and House or Senate votes, or be abandoned. New legislation could also be developed in the second session. All bills that did not make it to the Governor's signature by June 30, 2024, would have to be re-drafted in the next general assembly. Delaware would be electing a new Governor in November 2024, as Governor Carney completed his second term, which meant a new administration as well. Bills usually have a primary sponsor, an additional sponsor, and co-sponsors. Both senators and representatives can develop bills, and the more sponsors on each bill, the more likely the legislation will be approved. Also, bills with more sponsors generate media attention, which is the most likely way constituents hear about legislation. The state website has a search engine, and all bills are public information once they are released, but it requires a bill number, legislator name, or keyword to search. If the primary sponsor is a representative, the bill starts in a House committee; conversely, if sponsored by a senator, it starts in a Senate committee. Each committee has a different number of members, and majority voting to release from committee is required before moving to the next step. Public comment, usually two minutes per person, is only allowed during the committee hearing. The committee could recommend that the bill not move forward, ask for an amendment in order to release the bill (with or without another review), or approve it as written. Depending on the bill's content, including if a fiscal note is required to support implementation, the next step could be another committee or to the chamber floor for a vote. Bills are required to have a majority vote from committees in each chamber plus the chamber floors before the Governor's signature step.

Our main priority was to raise awareness of our organization. In January, I published the first monthly newsletter, focusing on introducing our mission, key pillars, and goals. I started an email distribution list with people I interacted with over the years, people I met in my local town hall meetings who were interested, and asked coalition members to forward it to their network. On January 17, we spent the day at Legislative Hall educating legislators and staff members about our mission statement, priorities, and sharing our testimonials. One of the coalition members reserved a table on the second floor, and we displayed pictures of our loved ones. We printed testimonials of our stories and copies of our monthly newsletter, which described our goals. By the end of the day, we handed out every copy we brought with us and heard stories from legislators as well as state staff members about issues their families experienced with care for seniors. In the afternoon, Senator Mantzavinos officially recognized our coalition on the Senate floor. He stated we would be partnering on legislation this session and to reach out to us if they would like more information. Based on the feedback we received, it was clear that major changes are needed both in the community and facilities to ensure quality care is provided to our loved ones.

Kent General meeting

On January 24, 2024, I worked up the courage to read the hospital notes from Memom's time in Kent General Hospital. I vividly recalled the events that happened during the hospital stay and how I felt each day but wasn't ready until then to know more. Part of me felt like I needed to have more closure and peace about the assisted living facility before I dove into learning more about the hospital process. I was making progress on forgiving those involved with Memom's care (or lack thereof) before the hospital admission through serving as a voice for others harmed in long-term care facilities. Timing is key for change, and it wasn't meant for me to know what happened before. It took me two days to read through the amount of documents we had on her twelve days in the hospital. I took notes and used tabs to mark critical information I wanted to reference in the future. Reading the documents, I was reliving the horrors of her life those twelve days. Picturing Memom tied by her hands and ankles because she was in excruciating pain was something no human should ever have to experience. I decided that even though it had been almost three years, I needed to find out if policies and training either were in place or would be developed to prevent this. On the afternoon of January 25, 2024, I called the patient advocacy department to file a complaint.

The patient advocate who answered the phone listened as I cried while explaining what I had just learned. She validated my pain and asked me to write a letter capturing key points. This time, I experienced no minimizing or invalidating of my perception of what went wrong. She didn't ask about Memom's age or factors leading up to the admission. I appreciated her honesty that there may not be a full investigation due to the length of time that had passed, but she promised to send my letter to the right people. In the letter, I made certain that my intent was to help future patients as well as to feel my pain was heard and validated. One nurse, Tyler, was exceptional in his care for Memom and interactions with me. I felt it was important to acknowledge his excellence as a model for other caregivers at the hospital. Here is the letter I sent:

January 25, 2024

To whom it may concern:

I am filing a complaint regarding my grandmother's hospitalization at Kent General Hospital from February 4, 2021 to February 16, 2021. You may be wondering why I waited so long to file a complaint but I was still processing the neglect she suffered in the assisted living facility. My grandmother, Mary Jones Barthelmeh, was admitted to your hospital due to a foot wound the assisted living let get beyond their level of care. We were locked out of the facility and some members of our family did not want my grandmother removed from there. She was admitted with a diagnosis of sepsis and MRSA. I was aware of some care issues and staff interaction issues from her hospitalization but this week I finally went through her medical files from the stay and found more. My grandmother was a nurse at the Hospital for the Chronically Ill until she retired at age 68 and fully embodied the spirit of a nurse her whole life. She even had a nurse's prayer on her prayer card.

1. *In her admission notes, I read it stated she had dementia. My grandmother never had dementia and had a clear mind. The sepsis infection can cause mental acuity issues but documenting an improper diagnosis of dementia can alter the care provided.*

2. *In her pain assessment scores she consistently stated "0 out of 10" from admission until the morning of February 11th where the pain assessment changed to "advanced dementia." A nurse found my grandmother's toe in bed the morning of the 10th. No documented pain medicine, including acetaminophen, was given until the evening of February 13th when she was started on morphine injections. How can someone not be in pain with sepsis raging through their body and their toe rotting off? Every reputable health organization documents sepsis as severely painful with whole body pain. My mother and I were asked to come to the hospital that day (despite previously being told we weren't allowed) and saw my grandmother thrashing her head and body, obviously in pain. Another common side effect is acute confusion. Was my grandmother assumed to have dementia because of her age rather than confusion from a terrible infection? In fact, in her last quarterly assessment at the assisted living on 12/8/20, my grandmother wrote "Life is good, hang on!" to show her mental capacity. Does that sound like someone who doesn't want to live or is confused?*

3. *When we arrived on the 13th, the nurse asked me and my mother how we could have my grandmother full code, not DNR. My grandmother put together her advanced directive with her lawyer since she knows how critical it is. We were told on the 12th the toe was able to be safely amputated and planned for surgery on the 15th. It was a huge shock for us to walk in, see my*

grandmother throwing her head around and screaming in pain, while a nurse discussed the advanced directive in an accusatory manner. She even mentioned when my grandmother was rolling her eyes that she was ready to go to heaven. My grandmother went to church every Sunday, sometimes twice, and I never once heard her say she was ready to go. She carried my brother's wedding invitation in her purse and never got to attend in June 2021.

4. *I read in the notes that my grandmother was physically restrained by her ankles and wrists from the evening of February 10th through the evening of February 11th. This was not communicated to our family. It seemed there was no thought as to why she might be violent. Maybe she was in excruciating pain because of sepsis and her toe falling off that morning. I can understand wanting to protect the patient and staff but want to know the policy on notifying the family of use of physical restraints.*

5. *The first weekend my grandmother was in the hospital the iPad for FaceTime was not available. Each day we were told staff forgot to charge it. Throughout the couple of days I was able to eventually visit, I saw plenty of staff on their personal phones, so why can't the iPad be charged?*

6. *We were told by a nurse my grandmother would likely die on February 14th. My mom, dad, and I were allowed to spend time with my grandmother that day. She did not die that day so the next day we called and my mom and I were told we could both visit. We went during the day since we were driving from Millsboro to Dover and it was icy. The roads weren't safe at night. When we got to the hospital to check in we were told initially we could not visit. The ICU nurse manager called the desk downstairs*

to speak with me. I was told "I was lucky I was able to see my grandmother the day before and that she was not actively dying today." I'm not sure if "actively dying" is a medical term but I don't recommend telling someone they are lucky when their grandmother is dying from neglect and definitely don't use the term "actively dying." My mother was allowed in while I had to wait in the parking garage.

7. *The only person in the experience who I would ever want to treat me or someone I cared about is Tyler in the ICU. If your staff was a replica of Tyler and his exceptional abilities as a nurse then you would never receive a complaint. He treated my grandmother as a human even as she wasn't awake. He believed patients could hear you as I believe so too and he didn't distinguish care based on them being awake or not. He asked me about my grandmother's life and truly listened. I am thankful that my grandmother's last day on earth was with Tyler as her caregiver. She would've loved talking with him.*

8. *When I walked into the ICU on Sunday, February 14th, I saw a nurse at the desk watching Netflix on her phone. I do not expect people to be in patient areas watching shows on their personal phone. I didn't care at the time because I wanted to see my grandmother but phones should be reserved for break times. There are lots of studies on the lack of anyone's ability to multi-task.*

C. S. Lewis wrote, "Integrity is doing the right thing, even when no one is watching." I believe if my family was allowed to be involved in the care of my grandmother both at the assisted living and at your hospital that she would not have suffered neglect or abuse. Locking families out created more harm than good.

Given the large amount of issues and poor decisions that led to my grandmother's painful death, I would like to focus on the following:

1. *I recommend a refresher on sepsis training. Providing no form of pain management for someone in sepsis is cruel and inhumane. Even acetaminophen is a form of pain management. Also, cover acute confusion as a symptom.*
2. *Ageism training- don't assume everyone in their 90s has dementia. Infections such as UTIs and sepsis can cause confusion.*
3. *What is your policy on using physical restraints? Do you notify family when this is used?*
4. *Training on interacting appropriately with families. Maybe Tyler can give the training since he exceeds at nursing and communication.*
5. *Training on multitasking and the dangers to patients of doing so. I can provide some studies if necessary.*

On the evening of February 16th, I held my grandmother's hand, told her all of my favorite memories with her, and told her if she needed to let go that I would be ok. She died a couple hours later. I know she would want me to pursue advocating for others in her honor, both as a patient and as a nurse. She was not ready to die and didn't need to suffer as she did. Even though it has been 3 years, I believe the examples are still relevant to cover with staff.

Thank you for taking the time to read this, investigate, and do better. I look forward to your response.

Sincerely,

Candace Esham

A Nurse's Prayer

Let me dedicate my life today
To the care of those
Who come my way.

Let me touch each one
With healing hands
And the gentle art
For which I stand.

And when tonight
When the day is done.
Oh, let me rest in peace
If I have helped just one…

On February 14, 2024, I received an email from the patient advocate stating that the Senior Director of patient advocacy and the nurse, Tyler, reviewed my letter and wanted to meet with me. This validation of wanting to discuss my concerns and hopefully focus on continuous improvement for future patients was a welcome relief. I proposed a meeting on either February 21st or 22nd in person. The Senior Director called me the morning of February 19th to confirm a meeting at 11 a.m. on Thursday the 22nd. He genuinely wanted to hear from me and was open to my feedback.

I believe Memom sends me signs through words on license plates. On my way from my parents' house to the hospital, I saw a license plate that said "nurse24." It made me smile to think about Memom's passion for nursing and the intent of my discussion at the hospital regarding poor and excellent nursing behaviors. The significance of the 24 didn't click with me until I got home later that evening. Memom was born in 1924, and it was the year 2024—a sign of a year of healing for me. When I got to the hospital lobby, the Senior Director greeted me and directed me to a conference room. Tyler was sitting in the room, and I gave him a big hug. My eyes started tearing up thinking about his compassion and comfort then, as well as how he made me feel three years ago. On the table were three copies of my letter, ready to be reviewed. I am grateful for the professionalism and attention paid to each of my points. We discussed the programs and initiatives in place to prevent other patients from experiencing what Memom went through. Even though it was almost three years later, I felt a sense of relief knowing the organization recognized improvements were needed and that they apologized.

Freedom of Information Act

The Freedom of Information Act, often referenced as FOIA, was established in 1967 to allow the public the right to request access to records from any federal agency. Each state implements its own version of the Act and may have certain documents that can't be requested. For instance, Delaware does not allow public access to emails of General Assembly members, even if they are only carbon copied on them. Later in my advocacy journey, in February 2024, I requested "communications between the assisted living facility and the state of Delaware" for several roles involved in the lockdown decision-making. I included the Department of Health and Social Services Secretary, the Department of Healthcare Quality Director and Deputy Director, the Division of Public Health Director and Deputy Directors, Healthcare Commission Director, and the Division of Services for Aging and Adults with Physical Disabilities Director. Just over six months after requesting the information, I received a 626-page document detailing the email discussions regarding the reopening plan, visitations, vaccine distribution, support person roles, and even state funding for communicative technology.

State Civil Money Penalty funds could be applied for specifically by assisted living facility administrators during the pandemic for communicative technologies and accessories such as iPads, Microsoft Surface, or Facebook Portal. According to the FOIA request, only nineteen facilities in Delaware applied for these tools to help families stay connected with their loved ones. Memom's facility did not apply nor mention this was a possibility. No applications by facilities were denied by state officials.

On Thursday, September 10, 2020, the assisted living facility Memom resided in received the "Reopening Plan Application Form." In this form, there is "support person guidance," which provides "considerations for identification and designation of a support person who, prior to visitor restrictions, was regularly engaged with the resident." Failure to comply with the reopening plan or support person guidance could result in fines according to the form, but it's unclear if any were enforced. During the time period of September through November 2020, I reached out to numerous state officials and assisted living facility administrators, begging to know when or how my family could visit Memom. At no point did the term "support person" come up in the discussions. In fact, the only mention of this is in the document I requested. Support persons would be allowed one to four hours of visitation per day in the facility. In the completed form by Memom's facility director on December 1, 2020, the visitation plan was left blank on each of the eight questions.

Based on this form and the actions of the facility administrators, visitation was not considered a priority, and state officials did not question the incomplete form.

In order to assist facilities with staffing issues, federal nurses were contracted with the Department of Health. In a State Health Operations Center (SHOC) call, the Division of Nursing Home Quality Assurance Commission director asked for an update on the utilization of these resources paid for by the state, and Kate Brookins of the Division of Public Health reported that the nurses had nothing scheduled with any long-term care facilities. These were VA nurses, and some facilities did not respond at all to the offer for help. Facilities also did not keep the National Guard resources in their staff for very long, yet often claimed staffing issues.

On January 26, 2021, during another call, a member of the Department of Health stated, "the federal government oversees distribution" of the vaccines. The confusion on who owns the vaccine distribution plan likely delayed seniors from receiving their vaccinations. This led to delays in allowing visitors as well. Also in the call, one facility administrator mentioned that recently a "man and wife spouses admitted together to her facility" and inquired, "if they can co-habitate" in a private room. The decision was made "off-line," but the scrutiny of the question implied there was a possibility the couple would be separated. Another administrator stated, "family members are upset with the isolation" and "he is watching residents decline due to a lack of visitations." Dr. Levy, a Department of Healthcare Quality employee, said to "wait for national guidance and data," despite several states opening up visitation months earlier. The documentation of meetings and emails regarding visitation, resource management, and the vaccine distribution process highlighted the lack of transparency with the families who were desperate to see their loved ones.

VISITATION PLAN
For visitation to be permitted the following requirements are established. Screening and additional precautions including social distancing, hand hygiene, and universal masking are required for visitors.
18. DESCRIBE THE SCHEDULE OF VISITATION HOURS AND THE LENGTH OF EACH VISIT
19. DESCRIBE HOW SCHEDULING VISITORS WILL OCCUR
20. DESCRIBE HOW VISITATION AREA(S) WILL BE SANITIZED BETWEEN EACH VISIT
21. WHAT IS THE ALLOWABLE NUMBER OF VISITORS PER RESIDENT BASED ON THE CAPABILITY TO MAINTAIN SOCIAL DISTANCING AND INFECTION CONTROL?
22. DESCRIBE THE ORDER IN WHICH SCHEDULED VISITS WILL BE PRIORITIZED
23. DESCRIBE THE OUTDOOR VISITATION SPACE TO INCLUDE THE COVERAGE FOR SEVERE WEATHER, THE ENTRANCE, AND THE ROUTE TO ACCESS THE SPACE
24. DESCRIBE HOW A CLEARLY DEFINED SIX-FOOT DISTANCE WILL BE MAINTAINED BETWEEN THE RESIDENT AND THE VISITOR(S) DURING OUTDOOR VISITS
25. DESCRIBE THE INDOOR VISITATION SPACE THAT WILL BE USED IN THE EVENT OF EXCESSIVELY SEVERE WEATHER TO INCLUDE THE ENTRANCE AND THE ROUTE TO ACCESS THE SPACE
26. DESCRIBE HOW A CLEARLY DEFINED SIX-FOOT DISTANCE WILL BE MAINTAINED BETWEEN THE RESIDENT AND THE VISITOR(S) DURING INDOOR VISITS

Joint Finance Committee Meeting February 20, 2024

On February 20, 2024, the Joint Finance Committee meeting for the Department of Health & Social Services was held at Legislative Hall. It was the third time I provided public comment but the first time I attended in person. My mom attended the meeting with me, and other coalition members planned to call in virtually to speak. After signing in on the clipboard, my mom and I sat in the front row, anxious to hear if elder care would even be brought up. In previous years, I was usually the only one to mention seniors, as most conversations were about other populations such as children. This was our first official public comment appearance as a coalition, and we shared our written speeches among members ahead of time to make the most out of our two minutes each. I also emailed the committee comments two days before the meeting with links and more data than I could cover in two minutes. The letter included details about the funding the skilled nursing facilities were supposed to receive and the information I learned from the letter from the Medicaid department.

As usual, the committee hearing began with a presentation by the DHCQ director on accomplishments, challenges, and budget requests. An alarming statistic of a 75 percent increase in individuals placed on the Adult Abuse registry shocked legislators. 2,888 reports of alleged abuse, neglect, mistreatment, or financial exploitation, an increase of 51% over the previous year, were investigated. After the presentation, a significant number of questions from legislators followed. I became hopeful changes would happen since attention was being given to seniors, especially those living in long-term care facilities. The increase in funding for long-term care facilities was discussed specifically by the chair of JFC. His mother lived in an assisted living facility, and he asked staff of the facility if they received raises. The director of health-care reform for the state explained, "It's hard to know exactly how the money will flow after we give it to the nursing homes." Additional questions arose about how we can guarantee frontline workers would receive increases. A representative discussed how the state invested the money thinking it would result in wage increases and challenged whether we were "lining the pockets" of owners. The director stated this was a valid concern, and the secretary of the division claimed facilities "can't survive without paying more money to those doing frontline work." Assisted living facilities were not included in the long-term care facilities receiving the money, but this was not clarified until later. The conversation continued to drive the message about the responsibility of state investments and questioned where the money would be spent.

Sitting in the audience, I knew the form had the capability of having specific requirements, but the public was not allowed to comment at the time. I had provided some of the answers to these questions in my written comment submitted two days before the meeting, but it didn't seem to have made a difference based on the discussion.

Another interesting aspect of the meeting included questions about home healthcare agencies. A senator brought up that her constituent applied for a business license to open a home healthcare agency over two years ago and has not received approval. His proposal was behind 24 other agencies even two years later. She mentioned these services would keep people out of nursing homes, which impacts the state budget. The same state surveyors who are behind on required skilled nursing facility inspections were responsible for reviewing home healthcare agency applications. In 2021, the state received 48 interested providers for home healthcare agencies, and in 2023, they received 94 applications. Another representative stated his constituent operated home healthcare agencies in other states and wanted to open one in Delaware but was also in the backlog. Workforce challenges were brought up by the secretary of the division, but it made me wonder why so many people would want to open a business if they didn't think it would be successful. There were no vacancies in surveyor positions, but overtime was offered. For the first time since I participated in 2021, the conversations around senior care generated about an hour of discussion, showing a shift in the importance of the issues surrounding it.

Public comment began with each speaker given two minutes, with no dialogue between legislators and constituents. I was second on the list, followed by my mom. Here were our verbal comments:

Good morning, my name is Candace Esham.

Lack of oversight in long-term care facilities by government agencies allows neglect and harm to continue. Without frequent surveys and timely complaint investigations, systemic issues continue to harm our loved ones. Most recent available data on the backlog shows Delaware's Division of Health Care Quality has about 1,500 complaints for nursing homes and assisted living facilities. It would take 2.5 years at the current rate with zero additional complaints to get through the backlog. The percentage of Assisted Living complaints investigated has been consistently below 30% since 2013, on average 22% from 2013 to 2021. This is not new since the pandemic. According to a federal report, Delaware was one of 10 states that failed to meet Medicare's performance threshold for timely investigation of high-priority nursing home complaints every year from 2011 to 2018.

We ask that you fully fund positions to address the backlog, ensure survey timeliness, and prevent a significant backlog in the future. We also request DHCQ report quarterly to Margaret Bailey's group on the number completed each quarter and the backlog.

In addition, while the Medicaid reimbursement for skilled nursing facilities has not been assessed since 2008, we recommend if money is given to facilities to address staffing issues that there is transparency on what specifically this money is used for as was discussed this morning. Facilities should be tracking their staff vacancy rate and staff turnover rate. If these facilities are given money for staffing purposes, these two metrics should be reported at a minimum to show the money is being effectively used. I also would like to add that I asked Representative Williams for the *report that talks about the metrics around the $10 million and she was able to provide that for me so I encourage you all to look at that as you will find that the quality metrics are not quantifiable in that report. There is a lot of opportunity to use that report to require a return on investment if you will and in my opinion that report could use some work. Thank you.*

Next, my mom followed with her comments:

Good morning, my name is Lucilla Esham.

On February 5, 2021, we filed a complaint with DHCQ after we saw the photo of my mom's severe foot wound in her Bayhealth General online chart after she was sent to the ER with a stage 4 foot wound untreated for five months. She died eleven days later from sepsis and MRSA. The investigation took 285 days and the 31-page final report documented the facility failed to ensure attention to her physical needs, failed to follow its policies for skin and wound care, and policies for when a resident has a change in condition. Despite my mother dying from these injuries, the complaint was not filed as "immediate jeopardy." The time lag left other residents susceptible to similar injuries or death.

According to DHCQ website, as of January 19, 2024, out of the total of 42 assisted livings in Delaware, only 18 have been surveyed in the last 15 months. 5 facilities have surveys older than 3 years and 5 facilities have never been surveyed.

Out of the total of 45 skilled nursing facilities in Delaware, only 27 are current with the CMS requirement of a survey at least every 15 months. Five facilities have surveys older than 3 years and 2 facilities require a professional monitor due to severe deficiencies.

We ask that you fully fund positions to address the backlog, ensure survey timeliness, and prevent a significant backlog in the future. We also request DHCQ report quarterly to Margaret Bailey's group on the number completed each quarter and the existing backlog. The true measure of any society can be found in how it treats its most vulnerable members. Let us rise to that measure.

Several more members of the public commented following our testimony, including the executive director of the Delaware Nursing Home Residents Quality Assurance Commission, the former director of the Division of Healthcare Quality, and industry representatives. Comments included an emphasis on the need for positions to ensure oversight of long-term care facilities, acknowledgment of the removal of staffing ratio requirements in the last budget bill, and repeated concerns about the inadequate frequency of surveys. The most traumatic testimony came from a member of the public who was a resident of a long-term care facility due to recovery from an attempted suicide. He said, "From the worst of things come the best of things." His experience was the best because he was informed and understood what his needs were and how to get out of the facility. The industry profits from beds, not people. In his three months as a resident, he realized no one knew the role of an ombudsman, and he couldn't imagine what would be reported if people knew their rights. "It's 11 o'clock, do you know where your parents are?" is an article he would write based on staff shortages at night, with one nurse covering rehabilitation and the long-term care facility. He described the lack of staff and said the industry had been "hijacked by what happened with COVID." Imploring the legislators to quit investing in the industry that only has profit in mind, he wanted to keep people in their homes.

Rehabilitation was a gateway to long-term care facilities. His testimony was the only firsthand perspective of care for residents in a facility and painted a clear picture of the state of affairs.

A director of the oldest non-profit facility in Delaware spoke about the funding and claimed, "those funds are long gone." He listed the financial incentives provided to staff, including contractors, and said the facility is "struggling to survive." Another director increased nursing salaries five times since 2020, offered annual raises, education reimbursement, and is still left with vacancies and turnover. The comments from industry representatives and other members of the public starkly differed. One focused on the viability of their businesses, while the other described neglect, lack of oversight, and concern for a vulnerable population. The meeting adjourned, and I reflected on the benefits of preparation for the meeting by investigating where last year's money went. I felt the momentum of advocates for quality care improvements shift and was proud of the questions legislators asked.

Long-term care bill package

I knew a package of bills focused on long-term care facilities would be released this session but didn't know the exact date it would be made public. Our coalition was having monthly meetings to discuss strategy and ways to have our voices heard. During our February 8th meeting, some members expressed concern over the current bills that had not made movement and questioned whether any other bills would be developed. I shared their worry due to how slowly the legislative process can move. Negotiations and drafting for the bills Senator Mantzavinos and Representative Johnson planned to sponsor was ongoing, and I couldn't discuss the details yet. I asked my team members to have faith and patience in the process as well as in me. Coalition members knew how cumbersome the legislative meetings were but trusted our proposal would make an impact. On Wednesday, February 21, 2024, I received a preview of the four bills in the long-term care package. A virtual press conference was planned for the following Monday, and I was asked to be a part of it. All local media sources were invited to attend, and the bills would be public information after the press conference. I couldn't believe I would have five minutes to cover our coalition and perspective on the importance of each bill. This was the first opportunity to formally introduce our group's mission to the media. It felt like investing all my time into advocacy and the coalition was paying off.

The four pieces of legislation aligned with two of our key pillars: transparency and accountability for all care services, and best-in-class care for residents at all facilities. Splitting the changes into four different bills rather than one would allow for amendments to be made more easily along the process. When too many modifications are included in one bill, opponents can justify vetoing the legislation due to concerns with one section. One of the bills originated in the House and three in the Senate. House Bill 300 required all assisted living facilities to maintain accreditation from an independent accrediting organization approved by the Department of Health and Social Services; facilities that provide dementia services must maintain certification from an independent accrediting organization and define dementia care services and secured dementia care unit in Delaware code. Dementia care units were not defined in Delaware code, which meant no oversight of these services. Both assisted living facilities and memory care facilities were expected to be managed by state regulations and had no federal oversight.

Several industries, including healthcare, education, and even nuclear power, developed accreditation processes to certify institutions against quality standards. In July 2021, The Joint Commission launched an accreditation program focused on assisted living facilities to help organizations implement best practices and improve care. This organization was well-known in the healthcare community for acute care standards, and all Delaware hospitals utilized their services. Accreditation of facilities provides a valuable external perspective of performance against nationally recognized standards. It provides a framework for facilities to develop strategies to address the most complex issues and identify key vulnerabilities in the resident care experience, according to The Joint Commission website. Long-term care facility owners in nine states and Washington, D.C., currently volunteered to use this process to ensure quality care. An assisted living facility in Missouri was the first to receive The Joint Commission's assisted living memory care certification. This facility consistently ranks among the top communities in the nation, as determined by the U.S. News & World Report's Best Senior Living ratings. It also obtained a Great Place to Work certification, and accreditation has helped with worker retention. Despite the documented benefits of this program, I expected this mandatory requirement for accreditation to be the most opposed bill by the industry representatives.

Senate Bill 215 amended Title 16 of the Delaware Code relating to state inspections of long-term care facilities to require inspections on an annual basis. Changing the survey frequency from "regular" to "annual" would provide better oversight of long-term care facilities. Without defined timing, "regular" could be open to interpretation. As discussed previously, legislators modified the language to less specific requirements in 2018. Senate Bill 216 increases the civil penalties for violations of statutes in Title 16, Chapter 11 related to long-term care facilities, including abuse, neglect, mistreatment, or financial exploitation of residents. The maximum civil penalty had not been increased since 2000. This bill also repealed the provision that placed a cap on the civil penalties for continuing violations. Senate Bill 217 created a professional loan-to-grant incentive program to encourage Delawareans to pursue careers in nursing at long-term care facilities. The professional loan-to-grant incentive program to encourage students to pursue careers in nursing at long-term care facilities serving our most vulnerable population will help build a pipeline of workers. As I heard in meetings over the years, workforce shortages dominated concerns expressed by industry representatives, and this bill provided state funding to assist with recruitment. In the press conference, I discussed Memom's love for her career as a nurse, especially at the Hospital for the Chronically Ill in Smyrna. Her residents frequently did not have family, and she made sure they all felt valued and received the best care. She became a nurse to fulfill her passion for serving others by attending Emory University nursing school through the WWII cadet nursing program.

The media coverage of the package established improvements to quality care for seniors as a priority for this legislative session. Our organization was mentioned in local TV evening news and each local newspaper. We saw an increase in Facebook activity for our coalition and gained momentum with more followers. With the release of the bills, our focus could shift to specifically reaching out to legislators for support and preparing for committee hearings. The timeline for next steps wasn't clear, but we knew the opposition to these bills would be strong based on years of advocating individually.

Federal Advocacy

Based on media coverage during the pandemic, elder neglect in long-term care facilities occurred nationally. No state seemed to have the right amount of oversight and systems in place to provide consistent quality care. Since Delaware has only one U.S Representative, we decided to focus our advocacy efforts on state level legislation but monitored federal activity. The Senate Special Committee on Aging, first established in 1961, studies issues and submits finding and recommendations for legislation to the Senate. On January 25, 2024, the U.S. Senate Special Committee on Aging held a hearing on assisted living facilities for the first time in 20 years. While there are currently no federal regulations for these facilities, long-term care trends are supposed to be reviewed by this committee. Articles published by The Washington Post, New York Times, and KFF Health News focused on the safety and costs of assisted living facilities, which prompted the hearing. "Understaffed and neglected: How real estate investors reshaped assisted living" by MacMillan and Rowland, published on December 17, 2023, in *The Washington Post*, described a Colorado assisted living facility resident dying "after banging repeatedly on the locked doors" of the facility in "subfreezing temperatures." Since 2018, over 2,000 people left facilities unsupervised, resulting in the death of 98 residents. A Delaware resident who died is included in this group. Profits seemed to be a focus for operators rather than quality of care. A law passed in Congress in 2008 "gave investors the ability to hold senior-housing properties tax-free while also taking a slice of their annual income." The article further detailed that investors "receive returns of nearly 9 percent a year on average – more than double the yield for offices and hotels." The media coverage highlighted failures in care and exorbitant costs to the families.

Senator Bob Casey's comments revealed that "nearly a million Americans live in more than 30,000 assisted living facilities across our nation." By 2050, "nearly one in four Americans will be 65 or older," according to Senator Mike Braun's statement. Representing Indiana, he mentioned that his state "requires staffing ratios, dementia training, and maintains a website that discloses reports and enforcement actions."

These actions aligned with what our coalition wanted in Delaware and provided us data for what other states already had in place. The hearing continued with testimony provided by an advocate, Patricia Vessenmeyer, whose husband had dementia and lived in an assisted living facility. Her experience echoed that of families in Delaware. She listed poor facility design, understaffing, and inadequate staff training as contributors to neglect. Patricia even told a story of saving a man's life. While visiting her husband, she "heard someone crying for help." When she ran into the hallway, she "found the old man on the floor, trying to prevent himself from being beaten with his own cane by another resident." It was several minutes before a staff member came to help. Others testified regarding recommendations, including national standards to improve transparency, quality, and accountability. The Committee requested that constituents email their stories to members for further investigation. Hearing traumatic reports from others across the nation and learning the staggering statistics proved how urgent systemic changes were needed.

Delaware Caucus on Aging

In an email I wrote to Representative Williams in February 2021, I suggested a state caucus for seniors. Three years later, on February 15, 2024, the first meeting for the Delaware Caucus on Aging was held. It took recommendations from two separate task forces, but finally, the resources were assigned to develop the caucus. Led by Senator Mantzavinos and Representative Johnson, the purpose of this caucus is to provide a forum for discussing issues impacting seniors and their caregivers. At each meeting, guest speakers present topics with stakeholders including legislators, members of the public, community-based care leaders, and long-term care representatives. According to the Delaware "Aging in Place" report published on April 29, 2022, approximately 19% of Delaware's population is 65 and over, emphasizing the large number of senior constituents. Both community-based and facility-based care are areas for discussion. In the February meeting, Melissa Smith, the Director of the Delaware Division of Services for Aging and Adults with Physical Disabilities, presented an overview of the services provided by the state. The key takeaway was that Delaware's aging resident population is growing exponentially, and systemic changes are needed in both community-based and institutional care to allow our residents to thrive. Based on the room full of people wanting to learn more and get involved, it was clear the caucus was important.

The March meeting helped me finally gain clarity on the financial impact of community care versus facilities. Director Andrew Wilson of Medicaid & Medical Assistance presented that for the fiscal year 2025, the Delaware state and federal budget for Medicaid was approximately four billion dollars. The entire state of Delaware budget was six billion dollars, and the one billion dollars of state funding for the Medicaid program was a significant investment of taxpayer money. Delaware, with a population of around one million people, had an estimated 270,334 enrollees in the program for fiscal year 2025. While eligible recipients included more than just seniors, the members receiving support for home and community-based and institutional services utilized a large portion of the budget. In fiscal year 2023, the state spent over $465 million on long-term supports for just under 12,000 seniors in their homes and facilities. Services for individuals using community-based support cost around $22,667 per year compared to $79,346 per year for institutional services. In other words, for every person in a skilled nursing facility, the state could support four to stay in their homes. Budget concerns dominated the media and conversations in legislative hall, and in this meeting, stakeholders were shocked at the amount of money spent on these programs. Reflecting on the discussion regarding the backlog of applicants for home health agency licenses, I asked the director if improving the timeliness of the approval process could help not only with the budget but with residents' desire to remain in their homes. He was unaware of the delay in approval and committed to following up with the division of healthcare quality. No data was provided on how many individuals were unable to receive adequate services at home, causing families to move their loved ones into a skilled nursing facility. However, people I spoke with over the years described the lack of availability of resources in the community. It seemed not only better to provide services to residents at home from a personal preference but also a fiscally responsible decision.

Staffing ratios

While our coalition was focused on state legislation, we were monitoring the media for details of a federal mandate for staffing ratios in skilled nursing facilities. Delaware established Eagle's Law in 2000, which included minimum staffing ratios per shift, and the newly proposed federal standard was less than what the state currently required. These requirements were waived during the pandemic until January 2025, but once reinstated, they are designed to protect residents and staff in facilities. Two current state representatives and one former published opinion pieces in local newspapers, objecting to the federal mandate. In the *Daily State News* on March 1, 2024, Representative Short claimed, "staff mandates for nursing homes would hurt patients." He also stated, "currently, 93% of our state's nursing homes do not meet the three requirements of the proposed rule," costing "$13 million annually for our state to hire the additional workers needed to meet it."

On March 14, 2024, Representative Hilovsky added, "actions need to be taken to avoid staffing mandates" in the *Daily State News*, emphasizing, "we shouldn't put our seniors and veterans in harm's way." At this point, no committee hearings were held for our state legislation, and I became worried the conversation about the need for adequate staff was shifting in the media. I wrote both representatives individually, and my own opinion piece was published on March 24, 2024, "Coalition disagrees about nursing home staffing mandates."

The Delaware Elder Care Advocacy Coalition was formed by families who promote legislation for Delaware aging residents to ensure they receive quality care and thrive. We are writing in response to both Representative Short and Representative Hilovsky's recent Opinion pieces in the Bay to Bay News. We are grateful for Representative Short's support on the 4 recent long-term care reform bills and Representative Hilovsky's support on one of the 4.

While we agree the workforce in the long-term care industry is challenged, we disagree that staffing ratio requirements "hurt patients." In these pieces, it was stated "nursing homes turn away new residents because they don't have enough staff." According to the Non-Acute Long-Stay Patient Task Force meeting on February 27, 2024, the 300 residents who are currently in acute settings who aren't able to be discharged due to placement issues and not due to staffing issues in Skilled Nursing Facilities. We encourage legislators to listen to the task force meeting and be involved with the members in the solution to moving these residents out of a hospital setting. Also, the DHSS Secretary was asked by Senator Sturgeon in the Joint Finance Committee hearing around 12:15 pm on February 20, 2024 are there residents waiting for those who are waiting for beds in skilled nursing facilities. The Secretary responded "it is typically not because there is not a bed available and typically a compounding factor. Those folks are stuck for other reasons." The reason residents remain in the hospital longer than needed for the level of care is not due to lack of beds in skilled nursing facilities. It is important to properly analyze the problem and causal factors before determining solutions or simply condemning legislation without providing a solution.

On February 26, 2024, Senator Mantzavinos and Representative Johnson released a four-bill package for long-term care reform. Senate Bill 217 is one of the bills and it focuses on creating financial assistance in the form of a professional loan-to-grant incentive program to encourage Delawareans to pursue careers in nursing at long-term care facilities. Enabling a workforce to invest in a career taking care of our most vulnerable population is critical. We encourage support on this bill.

There are several studies including the "Appropriate Nurse Staffing Levels for U.S. Nursing Homes" report that show a "strong positive relationship between the number of nursing home staff who provide direct care to residents on a daily basis and the quality of care and quality of life of residents." Another study conducted by an Institute on Aging noted the following relation-ship between Quality of Care Requirements and Nurse Staffing Requirements:

- *Insufficient nurse staffing levels, nursing staff without needed qualifications, and high nursing staff turnover rates contribute to inadequate care of residents.*

- *Staffing shortages, staff burnout, and lack of needed staff training contribute to mistreatment of residents.*

Lack of oversight and standards in long-term care facilities can cause grave danger to our most vulnerable populations. There have been several cases in our state in the last few years.

- *In February 2021, a resident of Dover Place died due to sepsis and MRSA from a wound beyond the level of approved care in an assisted living. The state investigation determined that for two of the three sampled residents, the facility failed to revise the service agreements when the needs of the residents changed.*
- *In May 2021, a resident of Courtland Manor in Dover, Delaware died from sepsis and organ failure. The lawsuit claims the nursing home staff failed to change the resident's catheter for more than a year.*
- *In February 2022, a resident of Newark Manor was found dead outside after she fell off the balcony. This facility was sued by the Attorney General's Office for long-standing issues from 2011 to 2017 including being under-staffed.*

These are only a few of the devastating stories of lack of care occurring in our state. We should not be condoning opening beds in facilities simply to have a physical place for residents to stay without requiring these facilities to ensure quality care is provided, especially when lack of beds isn't typically the cause for long-term hospital stays.

In addition, skilled nursing facilities are not the only option for discharge from the hospital. Home health care agencies are options to provide care in the comfort of their own home.

*However, there is a two-year backlog on business owners wait-
ing for the application process with the Delaware Division of
Healthcare Quality as discussed in the Joint Finance Committee
hearing. Last year, there were 94 interested providers for new
home health care agencies.*

*The state has established a Caucus on Aging, led by Senator
Mantzavinos and Representative Johnson. The next meeting will
be held on Thursday, March 28, 2024 from 10:30 am to 12 pm
in the Tatnall Building, Room 112. Director Andrew Wilson of
Medicaid & Medical Assistance will be the guest speaker. For
more information, please contact Brandon Williams at BrandonF.
Williams@delaware.gov. We encourage legislators to join the
conversation in understanding the problems and working to
provide solutions in our state to ensure our aging residents thrive.*

Senate Health & Social Services Committee Hearing- No bull

Four weeks passed since the release of the long-term care bill
package before the first committee meeting occurred to discuss them.
Several coalition members wrote to every senator and representative
asking for support for the bills in the meantime. The initial step in the
approval process for two of the four bills was the Senate Health &
Social Services hearing on Wednesday, March 27, 2024. Senate Bill
215 modified the survey frequency, and Senate Bill 216 increased the
amount for civil money penalties. I learned of the meeting a few days
before the date the bills would be heard and made sure to share the
information with my coalition members. We planned for a united front
in the meeting.

Over the weekend, I opened every posted state survey for all skilled nursing facilities and assisted living facilities. The state department of healthcare quality uploads the surveys on their website for transparency of the services provided and findings. My family used survey findings and complaints to determine which facility we thought Memom would be the safest in Dover. The state director stated they were almost caught up with surveys at a meeting in February, but this was not updated on the website. Historical surveys are not available unless a "Freedom of Information Act" request is submitted, which takes time and can potentially cost hundreds of dollars. I didn't know how many of the surveys had been completed and not uploaded, so I decided to reference the publicly available information in my speech and in written comments to the committee members. In the email, I provided a table with each facility's name and last posted survey date if over a year in a table.

In my review, I found incidents of everything from resident harm, neglect, and abuse to incidents where staff did not receive proper support to do their jobs. I needed to convince the committee of the benefit of survey timeliness for oversight of resident and workforce safety, and each report confirmed this importance. It was clear after reading several surveys that there was a theme of staff training not being conducted, issues with reporting injuries to the state, and an overall lack of adherence to standards. Investigations identified the quality concerns and required agreement between surveyors and the facilities on corrective action plans to prevent reoccurrence. With the information available, it seemed obvious that the regulation change was important, but I knew it would generate pushback based on years of advocacy.

I made sure I arrived at the Senate chamber for the hearing 30 minutes early, as another bill in the hearing had significant support from hospitals in Delaware. There are limited seats around the outside of the Senate chamber, and securing one for the two-hour meeting was important to have access to speak. Even though I arrived early, there were only two chairs left. Having spoken at several state meetings over the years, I knew most of the people who would make comments. As I was signing in for public comment, I saw two people who had been advocates for better long-term care for years and went over to share my excitement about the bills with them. Not every bill gets heard in committee if it isn't a priority for multiple legislators. The most important part of planning for the speech was predicting any contradictory evidence or doubts legislators might have regarding supporting the bill. By anticipating what the opposition would say to challenge the bill, I could include facts to counter their position. In previous years, when I focused on Memom's story only rather than the bigger picture, I was not successful in convincing others that change was needed.

Two amendments to the bills were published on the state website the night before to accommodate feedback from stakeholders. I was familiar with the possibility of amendments to bills from my professional work experience but hadn't realized timing could be so close to the hearing date. Originally, Senate Bill 215 changed the survey frequency from "regular" to "annual," but the amendment changed the frequency to "mirror requirements in federal regulations," which are annually but no longer than every 15 months. The federal regulations only applied to skilled nursing facilities, not assisted living or dementia-care services, but the intent was to give a 3-month grace period for Delaware long-term care facilities. State regulations would cover all long-term care facilities. This slight modification still met the oversight changes needed and would provide less confusion between state and federal frequency requirements. Also, the implementation date was changed.

Over an hour passed discussing other bills before Senate Bill 215 was presented. A fiscal note of $800,000 was required to support the survey frequency change. With ongoing pressure to reduce the state budget, funding was questioned even though committee members recognized the importance of the surveys. Overall, the committee members spoke in favor of the bill. When public comment started, the first person, former director for the Division of Healthcare Quality, stated her support for the bill but expressed "major concerns." She recalled resources were only funded by the federal government for facilities covered by CMS, skilled nursing facilities. State-licensed facilities did not receive survey funding. In one of my previous roles, I assisted departments in a major healthcare system with staffing models. I knew if there wasn't a requirement to perform a task, in this case a survey, then resources would not be allocated to perform the work. Also, the purpose of the legislation was for survey timing, not how the department would assign resources. This bill added the requirement and the funding for personnel or contract services, so I didn't understand the concern. In the JFC meeting, the director said no positions were open for surveyors, conflicting with comments from speakers. Another state employee provided recommendations to develop a "robust training program" for surveyors and timely posting of surveys. When it was my time to speak, I focused on the merits of the bill specifically, rather than other challenges to the oversight system.

Good morning. My name is Candace Esham, founder of the Delaware Elder Care Advocacy Coalition.

Changing survey frequency from "regular" to mirror requirements in federal regulations will provide better oversight of long-term care facilities. According to the DHSS website, one skilled nursing facility has not been surveyed since 2017 with 14 out of 47 over a year since surveyed. For assisted living, 4 facilities do not have surveys available, and one has not been surveyed since 2011. 30 of 43 have not been surveyed in over a year.

Quality care and fiscal responsibility go hand in hand. Holding facilities accountable when standards are not maintained should prevent longstanding, systemic issues. Examples of recent findings in Delaware long-term care facilities are:

- *For 6 out of 16 sampled staff members, the facility failed to ensure that staff received initial or annual Emergency Preparedness training.*
- *Failure to immediately report an allegation of abuse to the administrator.*
- *For 3 out of 16 sampled staff members, facility failed to ensure required trainings on abuse, neglect, exploitation, and dementia management were completed.*
- *Failure to report falls with injury to the State Agency as required.*
- *Failure to ensure 3 out of 6 residents reviewed for abuse were free of sexual abuse by another resident with a history of sexually inappropriate behavior.*
- *A delay of 15 days in communication with orthopedics to change treatment order after wound care identified a boot was exacerbating the pressure wound.*

These surveys are important to ensure safety issues are documented, root causes performed, and corrective actions developed as well as giving residents and families data to make informed decisions before choosing a facility. It is not only a safety matter for residents but ensures the operators of facilities enable their staff to provide better care.

Senator Mantzavinos presented Senate Bill 216 after the public comment ended for SB 215. Civil penalties are enforced when long-term care facilities violate a standard. The value of penalties had not been increased since 2000 and needed to be adjusted based on inflation. Comments from some members of the public focused on details outside of the intent of the bill, including developing a rubric for penalties, interfering with investigations, and a reduction in penalties if the facility does not challenge the penalty. It seemed as if others wanted to solve a multitude of issues with the process rather than just increasing the fines. I heard several legislators say "progress over perfection" regarding legislation over the last few years and believed moving forward with some improvements in the right direction was better than nothing. My goal was to reveal the types of neglect occurring in facilities throughout Delaware.

Good morning, again. According to the Division of Healthcare Quality, in 2023 there was a 75% increase in the individuals placed on the Adult Abuse registry. Also, 2888 reports were investigated of alleged abuse, neglect, mistreatment or financial exploitation of seniors last year. These two data points show it is more critical now than ever to provide oversight to all long-term care facilities.

Lack of oversight and inadequate penalties for violations in long-term care facilities can cause grave danger to our most vulnerable populations. A few examples are:

- *In February 2021, my own grandmother died due to sepsis and MRSA from a wound beyond the level of approved care in an assisted living. The state investigation determined failure to meet the needs of other residents as well.*
- *On Christmas day 2021, a resident pushed another resident, causing her to break her hip. She died one month later. This facility had the highest number of reported abuse incidents in the state in the past decade.*

- *In May 2021, a resident died from sepsis and organ failure. The lawsuit claims the nursing home staff failed to change the resident's catheter for more than a year. The last survey was done September 2022.*
- *In August 2023, video footage revealed a resident being physically and verbally abused by staff. While putting the resident to bed, one staff member forcefully pulled the resident up in the bed and another staff member slapped the left leg of the resident. Their foot was grabbed, toes bent down forcefully, and staff member called the resident "a devil from hell." The other staff member laughed in the background. The last survey was done November 2021.*

Please pass SB 215 and 216. As the fastest aging state in the nation, we should strive to be a leader in providing exceptional care for our residents.

My comments were followed by a few long-term care industry representatives. A concern for the lack of increase in government funding for care, the cost of federal non-compliance fines, and a challenge to the tie to quality were brought up. It was claimed that facilities do a lot of self-reporting on incidents. No specific data was provided in the comments. One director stated these bills "painted the assisted living industry with a broad stroke, a wide brush just demonizing providers, and we are punishing the group for a few reported unhappy residents and families." Senate Bill 216 is "another example of the assisted living industry being in the crosshairs of legislation; punishing the group to appease those who have a bullhorn." He further went on to say, "hearing these horror stories is odd." Senator Mantzavinos followed up the public comments specifying the intent of this bill is for the values of penalties and other aspects of current law could be looked at in another bill. I left the meeting not knowing if either bill would receive committee approval. Delaware Senate Committee meetings do not publicly vote during the meeting and the results are posted online later. House Committee meetings usually have a roll call with votes at the end, so it is clear the fate of the bill. Feelings of happiness for the bills making it to the first step of the process were tainted with anger and disgust from some of the public comments. As I turned right on Legislative Avenue to head home, I saw a license plate with the words "NO BULL." Reflecting on the speech from the director regarding people who have a bullhorn, I laughed at what I perceived as a message from Memom to keep fighting.

Proverbs 28:1 "The wicked flee when no man pursueth: but the righteous are bold as a lion."

One of the bills in the long-term care package, House Bill 300, focused on accreditation and defining dementia care in the state of Delaware code. In the first Caucus on Aging meeting, held in February 2024, an executive director for an assisted living facility in Delaware casually mentioned that the industry could not afford to have one more regulation. This sentiment was echoed in the comments given by industry representatives in the Senate Health & Social Services Committee hearing. The original intent of House Bill 300 was to require all assisted living facilities to maintain accreditation from an independent accrediting organization approved by the Department of Health and Social Services. The state, rather than the federal government, regulated assisted living facilities, and the accreditation process would provide a forum to utilize best practices from other states. This would save state resources from having to research regulations and outcomes since the accrediting organization performs those tasks. I knew this bill would be the most challenged as Delaware would be the first state mandating accreditation for licensed facilities. However, as facilities in nine other states and D.C. volunteered to participate in the program, I thought reaching out to management in other states that decided to invest in accreditation might help.

The Joint Commission is an organization that specializes in the accreditation of several types of healthcare specialties. In July 2021, they launched a program specifically for assisted living communities to provide consistent and reliable care for residents. According to their website, they recognized these communities have been "increasingly shifting from a mostly hospitality-based environment to a more health-care-focused setting by offering services for medication management, skilled nursing, and dementia care." They developed standards with a team of experts to "design standards that align with quality care delivery and safe practices." Five standardized performance measures are tracked and reported: off-label antipsychotic drug use, resident falls, resident preferences and goals of care, advanced care plan/surrogate decision-maker, and staff stability. I was familiar with the benefits of accreditation in my roles as an engineer in the nuclear power industry and as a performance improvement specialist in an acute care hospital setting. Both industries required accreditation to ensure quality standards were shared and implemented. While researching the program on The Joint Commission website, I came across an article with an interview with an executive director of a facility that maintained accreditation and wanted to know more about their decision to do so.

On Friday, March 29, 2024, I Googled the facility and called their hotline number. I asked the receptionist if the executive director was available to speak to me about the accreditation process. Much to my surprise, I was connected to him, and he offered to share his insights. I explained the mission of my coalition and the bill requiring accreditation. When I described Memom's story and other neglect tragedies, he expressed his sympathy and stated the industry must do better not only because it is the right thing to do but for viability as a business. I shared the opposition to the bill and asked for ideas on how to convince facility administrators of the benefits of the program. He explained his facility did not have to invest in a lot of new programs because they already had robust training and fall prevention strategies, for example. However, he said if facilities were poor performers, then it would be a struggle for them to achieve accreditation. Quoting Proverbs 28:1, "The wicked flee when no man pursueth: but the righteous are bold as a lion," he emphasized the outspoken opponents likely have major quality issues in their facilities. While he didn't have ideas for ways to convince facilities to adopt the program, he did provide meaningful insight into the urgency to provide better care and how his residents, staff, and even profits improved after implementation. In early April, I emailed every state representative and senator, asking for support for the bill and shared a summary of the discussion I had with the executive director, hoping to prove the value of it from the industry perspective. Only one representative wrote me back, expressing support.

House Health & Human Development Committee
Meeting Wednesday, April 24, 2024

Almost a month passed between my conversation with the executive director regarding accreditation and the hearing for HB 300. Most of my communications before this hearing were with the Senate side of legislators, and typically, I received a text or email a couple of days before any meeting from a staff member. Unfortunately, there was a gap in communication between me and House staff. The morning of Wednesday, April 24, 2024, I received a phone call from Representative Johnson asking if I was aware HB 300 would be heard in committee today. I panicked, thinking I missed an email or notification, but we both realized the gap in communication. During the call, I reminded Representative Johnson of the research I did with another facility and an accreditation organization, as well as stressed the importance of emphasizing that everyone wins with quality care. As soon as I got off the phone, I texted my coalition team members, hoping many could join with testimony despite the short notice. I had no idea about the availability of group members and if they would have their thoughts put together for the potential two-minute maximum public comment period. None of us lived close enough to get to Legislative Hall in an hour. Eighty minutes later, legislators would be discussing the merits of requiring accreditation for assisted living facilities. Luckily, I prepared my speech a few days after the discussion with the director in another state, but I knew speaking in person would be more powerful. If bills have significant discussion by legislators and a large turnout of in-person comment, virtual comments can get cut short or even eliminated.

I registered for virtual comment and logged onto the Zoom meeting a few minutes before it began. When the meeting formally started, I could see the outer chairs around the room full of long-term care facility lobbyists and only one person who I thought might advocate for the bill. My heart sank thinking about how many minutes of comment time opposers to the bill would have. Hopeful for minimal legislator discussion, I quickly found out how wrong I was. Several members of the committee were absent, but a quorum was met, so the meeting officially began. Representative Johnson presented the bill as a recommendation from the long-term care task force from the previous year due to inconsistent standards of care and a growing number of instances in which residents of Delaware's assisted living facilities have been subjected to substandard care that has threatened their health and safety. Assisted living facilities are not subjected to federal regulations nor to any regulations related to providing memory care services. She discussed the cost as provided by the Joint Commission as $4,000 to $5,000 annually and an additional fee of $6,500 every three years when the survey is conducted. She spent her entire career serving vulnerable populations and has seen how dignified care can improve an individual's quality of life, setting forth a path of care holistically. In her introduction to the bill, she stated, *"For too long, we have heard news reports that strike fear in those with families in assisted living facilities... A lot of questions related to this legislation have been swirling around, opposition, emails, the why's... The current system we have is already voluntary."* She added that people claimed Delaware should not be the first to require accreditation. New Jersey passed legislation like this and challenged why Delaware can't be the first state to implement it. Delaware is small but aging rapidly. She mentioned that the bill closes the gap with state surveys, but this bill actually focuses on a proactive approach to best practices rather than reacting to a tragedy with a plan of correction. Representative Baumbach was the first to comment, acknowledging the criticality of the issue and how important the population is. Expressing concern, he challenged the method of achieving higher standards and "letting ourselves off the hook" by not requiring the state to have standards. Families are cash-strapped, and the implementation doesn't cost the state anything. Facilities will pass the costs along to families and residents. He acknowledged research, but he feared that if we shut down one facility, the state won't have a safe place for them. Ironically, he mentioned a quote: "If you want to see someone's priorities, see how they spend their money," and instead of showing that facilities don't want to spend their money on performance improvement for their residents and workforce, he described a "lose-lose situation."

"We will all lose if we do nothing. As it stands, we are not doing enough," Representative Johnson responded. Paying extra for a sense of relief for having appropriate oversight is something families would want. Two divisions, disabilities and behavioral health, in the state already require accreditation. Next, Representative Jones-Giltner, a retired nurse who attended the health portion of the Joint Finance Committee, recalled the department claiming surveys have not been the priority and that there are no open positions. I knew the survey process had a different intent than the performance improvement aspect of accreditation but had to listen to the debate without providing input. Seniors who live in an assisted living facility wrote to Representative Jones-Giltner about concerns, specifying that the level of care is appropriate for them. Representative Heffernan stated a facility in her district is "strapped for staff and costs" and expressed concerns about it closing if this bill was implemented. As legislators continued to discuss, I couldn't believe how many received letters in opposition to the bill and wondered what information was provided to the constituents to cause the fear of the bill. Acknowledging the fear, Rep. Johnson stated the "intent is for all of us to win. Think about how accreditation can change our services in a positive way."

Representative Morrison thanked Representative Johnson for her work on the long-term care task force but brought up costs associated with the requirement. High standards of care and continuous quality improvement cost money. If we all believe all our assisted living facilities are operating at the level they ought to be, accreditation only signifies great service. In her experience, there were no standards that were above what the state of Delaware required that hurt the facility's bottom line. It was elevating the quality of services. Conversations continued for over an hour, and it became clear no representative was in full support of the bill as written. A facility administrator was called upon as an expert witness to help answer a question, and I only wondered if I could've been called on to explain my research if I had been present in the room.

The chair of the committee promised public comment would not be cut shorter than two minutes. Six industry representatives used phrases such as "a barrage of bills aimed at assisted living," "unintended consequences," diverting facility resources, leading to facility closures, claims of the state "giving up their own laws," and the cost to residents when commenting on the bill. These remarks starkly contrasted with those of the director I spoke with, and I reflected on his message of "the righteous are bold as a lion." Fear dominated the concerns of legislators and others. Even the director of the Delaware Nursing Home Residents Quality Assurance Commission asked for the bill not to be released, citing that accreditation isn't the best solution and concerns with the fees. The only in-person advocate for the bill was the Delaware Director of Government Affairs of the Alzheimer's Association. By the time in-person comment ended, there was little time left in the meeting, and virtual public comment would be limited to one minute. I was the first to speak and had no time to cut my speech in half.

> *Good morning, my name is Candace Esham, founder of the*
> *Delaware Elder Care Advocacy Coalition. We support this bill.*
> *My grandmother died a painful death from neglect in an assisted*
> *living and I would have gladly paid more money to prevent*
> *that. Recently I spoke with an executive director at a facility*
> *in Missouri regarding the benefits of becoming accredited. His*
> *facility consistently ranks among the top communities in the*
> *nation as determined by the US News and World Report's Best*
> *Senior Living Ratings. It also obtained a Great Place to Work*
> *certification and accreditation has helped with worker retention.*
> *He noted investing in training of staff as required in the accredita-*
> *tion process not only provides quality care for residents but*

makes their employees feel valued. There are also cost savings in liability insurance. We hope the industry in Delaware embraces performance improvement and learning best practices to provide a better environment for their residents and workforce.

Several of my coalition members followed me in the virtual comment, imploring support for the bill. Each person cited the cultural issues with the industry and the lack of solutions provided by facility representatives. "They don't want you to shine the light," as told by a coalition member, perfectly captured our collective feelings. Just by not being in person, our voices were dampened and our messages shortened. The meeting concluded with Representative Johnson offering to speak with legislators and changing the mandatory requirement to voluntary for the bill to be released by committee. Even with this change, some representatives voted for the bill to not move forward. Not enough members were present to determine the outcome during the meeting. I left the call feeling defeated and frustrated that the information I spent hours researching was not considered.

Meetings for Amendments

Two bills from the spring 2023 legislative session sponsored by Senator Mantzavinos required negotiations with legislators, industry, and state stakeholders before being presented again to the Senate Health & Social Services Committee. Introduced on June 1, 2023, Senate Bill 150 defined dementia care services and activity services, required all long-term care facilities to have sufficient staff, and required staff training for dementia care. Originally, the bill required all staff to complete 12 hours of initial dementia care services training. The initial bill generated significant discussion during the June 14, 2023, committee hearing. Concerns around defining sufficient staff, which is language from CMS guidelines, enforcement of non-compliance, and confusion with regulations were expressed by several legislators. By specifying all long-term care facilities, skilled nursing facilities and assisted living facilities were included, which complicated the discussion of who defines regulations. It was clear during the hearing that the nuances of who provides oversight and the regulations governing standards were not understood. During public comment, seven industry representatives dominated the conversation, saying they were "an industry in crisis," facilities were "underfunded," and training would pull resources from direct care. Our coalition was not formed yet, and only one family member spoke in support of the bill. She explained the lack of regulations in assisted living facilities and dementia care units, answering some of the questions from earlier in the meeting. The meeting ended with the bill not moving forward, a legislator asking to be removed from sponsorship, and it being tabled until discussions between stakeholders occur in April 2024.

Stakeholders were invited to a private meeting to negotiate the language of SB 150 on April 25, 2024. Before the meeting, I researched the opposition to the bill by listening to the hearing recording from spring 2023 and reviewing requirements from other states regarding dementia care staffing and training. The meeting took place at Legislative Hall, and other invitees included me, the Executive Director of the Delaware Nursing Home Resident Quality Assurance Commission (DNHRQAC), the Delaware Director of State Government Affairs at the Alzheimer's Association, six industry representatives, and staff members supporting Senator Mantzavinos. Still disappointed and angry from the negative reaction in the meeting about the accreditation requirement from the day before, I planned to read the nurse's prayer and remind everyone of the human lives impacted by neglect, driving the need for change. Unless the attendees happened to read Memom's story in the newspaper from the previous spring, they didn't know my personal motivation for improvements. Two-minute speeches do not allow for a description of the suffering Memom experienced nor the grief I carried daily. When the meeting began, we were limited to an introduction of our names and organizations. Once again, I felt outnumbered and prepared for the bill content to be picked apart. The meeting lasted almost two hours, with most of the conversation driven by industry representatives. One industry leader referenced resident families' "perceived unhappiness" with care, causing these new regulations. I didn't respond and thought of how many horror stories I had been told over the years. By the end of the meeting, the bill contents had been weakened to only include assisted living facilities, excluding training requirements for residents with dementia in skilled nursing facilities, and requiring only four hours of initial training for direct care staff and two hours for non-direct care staff rather than the original twelve hours. I tried to focus on progress in moving the bill forward rather than the battle against change, but the lack of solutions provided by the industry to improve the quality of care overwhelmed me. Senator Mantzavinos remained committed to the bill and negotiating the terms even though long-term care stakeholders were challenging it.

The second bill from the spring of 2023, Senate Bill 151, initially required all long-term care facilities that provide dementia care services to complete a standardized disclosure form to protect against consumer fraud. Dementia care wasn't currently defined in Delaware code and, therefore, did not require specific licenses for care. The intent was for families to be able to use the form to compare facility services, including staffing plans, training, resident activities, policy on the use of psychotropic medication, and cost details. Similar legislation passed in

Texas in 2015. Some Delaware residents paid $16,000 per month out of pocket for institutionalized dementia care, and it wasn't always clear what services they should receive. No industry representatives were present to comment on the bill when it was discussed in the Senate Banking, Business, Insurance, & Technology Committee on June 7, 2023. Only the director from the Alzheimer's Association spoke and was in favor of the bill. Even though the bill received the number of votes required to be released from the committee, a stakeholder meeting was held on April 30, 2024. The same people who attended the previous week's Senate Bill 150 meeting were invited. One of my coalition members went to the meeting in my place as I was out of state on vacation. I joined the call virtually, but having a representative in person would ensure our coalition's voice would be heard more strongly. Once again, the industry representatives dominated the conversation with reasons why the bill was burdensome and would harm their business. The coalition member who attended the meeting had experience with neglect in dementia care services in a skilled nursing facility. His mother was a resident of a "secured memory care unit" and fell three stories off the balcony of a fire escape. She was found dead outside the facility, and it is still unclear how she was able to leave the "secured" area. During the meeting, he explained his personal experience and the importance of this bill to families. The negotiations continued for three hours. After the debate, only assisted living facilities would be required to comply, and the facilities no longer had to publish the disclosure on their website. Families would be provided a copy of the disclosure agreement, and the facility must submit a copy to the Department of Healthcare Quality. Despite the challenges from the industry, I admired Senator Mantzavinos' commitment to the bill and the dire need for improvements. The amendment to the bill did not require another review by a Senate committee and could move forward to a Senate floor vote.

May Movement

With the negotiations between stakeholders completed, the bills were ready to be heard in various committees and on the chamber floor. Between May and June, there were only seventeen days of session, and we could not afford any delays or backward movement in the bills if there was hope for them to pass this session. I included updates in the monthly newsletter and frequent Facebook posts, asking constituents to write their legislators in support of the bills. At this point, I was traveling to Legislative Hall at least once a week to speak and could feel the support from staff in the building. After I spoke in favor of Senate Bill 216, the bill to increase civil penalty values, even the security guard in the room asked to see a copy of my speech. He was shocked at the neglect happening and wanted to know more information. Awareness and education about the issues seemed to be making the most difference in support for the bills. Senate Bills 150 and 151 each received unanimous bipartisan support in the Senate floor meeting. During this meeting, there was no public comment allowed and minimal discussion of concerns about the bills.

SB 151- House Economic Development/ Banking/ Insurance & Commerce Committee, June 11, 2024

Good afternoon, my name is Candace Esham, founder of the Delaware Elder Care Advocacy Coalition. We support SB 151. When families are facing the difficult decision to put their loved one with dementia in an assisted living facility, they deserve to understand the services included in the care and consumer information on the facility. Disclosure requirements empower consumers by allowing families to compare facilities, receive clarity on any services that may be extra charges, and hold facilities accountable to meeting their claimed services. The most common statement I receive from families is they assumed dementia care training would be provided to all staff members. One of the disclosure requirements will be a description of the training plan. Other common concerns are surprised extra fees for services once their loved one is moved in such as for an aide. Established in 2015 in Texas, the disclosure statement promotes autonomy, innovation, and competition at the facility level. Other states with this requirement include California, Illinois, Minnesota, Rhode Island, and Tennessee.

Delaware is ranked as 10th most expensive state for memory care at a median monthly cost of $7,704, yet families do not always know what services they will receive or know what questions to ask. Some facilities cost up to $16,000 per month out of pocket in Delaware. Especially with the significant cost of care, families need to be able to compare facilities. People with dementia are a vulnerable population, requiring special care. This bill is a step towards transparency for safer, quality care for residents of facilities and a safer work environment for the staff who serve them. Let's join the states who have prioritized the need for dementia care disclosure requirements. We hope you support this. (Source: "How Much Does Memory Care Cost? A Complete State-by-State Guide" published on May 1, 2024 on A Place For Mom https://www.aplaceformom.com/caregiver-resources/articles/cost-of-memory-care)

Our coalition was awarded the 2024 Lt. Governor's Wellness

Challenge Community Spotlight Winners. Each year, the Delaware Lt. Governor accepts nominations for organizations that drive policy, system, and/ or environmental changes to improve the health of Delawareans. In March 2024, well before I knew how much progress we would make with legislation, I submitted an application describing the coalition's mission and initiative's sustainability, reach, and impact. Ten organizations throughout the state received the Community Spotlight award. During the awards ceremony on May 29, 2024, we learned about the organizations in our category. All other award winners had established non-profit status or some other funding source and some had over one thousand volunteers involved. With only nine core team members, I felt immensely proud of our group and the impact we were making. It was the end of May and none of our bills were ready for Governor signature. However, with the award and recognition from the second in command leader for Delaware, we remained hopeful at least one bill would pass.

June- The final month

In the month of June, there were only eight days of session. The first week had meetings for the Joint Finance Committee and there was also a holiday in this month. Eighteen separate votes across several meetings had to occur to get the six bills approved by June 30th. We could not afford any delays or setbacks if the bills were going to be approved. I spoke six times, all in person except one, to advocate for the bills. As session went on, family advocates, including members of my coalition, began to outnumber the industry representatives during public comment. We were well versed in our messaging, and it was clear we were determined to succeed. Even though industry representatives were involved in the negotiations for amendments, a few still expressed challenges to the bills during public comment. Legislators in committee hearings still had significant discussion on the challenges, especially with Senate Bill 150, the bill for dementia care staffing and training. Representative Johnson reminded them this bill was not a "fix-all" but a "tool in our toolbox." This sentiment reflected the mantra I learned, progress over perfection. In my professional experience in regulatory roles in the nuclear power and chemical manufacturing industry, I knew one bill or regulation would not solve all problems. Legislation was an iterative process and required stakeholders to be engaged with a solution mindset to be effective. Despite Representative Johnson's thorough explanation of the intent of the bill, a representative commented that senior care is an "impossible topic that is impossible to solve." At this point, I had attended over a dozen meetings this session where other bills were discussed, and I had never heard a legislator claim a problem was "impossible to solve." Regulations attempting to impact the opioid epidemic, aid children in foster care, institute human composting, and address dog barking laws received support without claims of impossibility. The lawyer who assisted in developing the bill was present to clarify the concerns with implementation, allowing the bill to be released from committee.

SB 150- House Health & Human Development Committee, June 12, 2024

Good morning, my name is Candace Esham, founder of the Delaware Elder Care Advocacy Coalition. We support SB 150. Current assisted living regulations for Delaware do not provide specifics around the staffing plan and training policies other than a requirement to have them. There are no requirements for the number of hours, frequency, or content of the training for staff.

Only Certified Nursing Assistants are required to have 6 hours of dementia training during each 24 month certification period.

Delaware is ranked as 10th most expensive state for memory care at a median monthly cost of $7,704, yet we do not have specific requirements for dementia care training. Some cost up to $16,000 per month in Delaware. "High-quality dementia care training can lead to an improvement in communication between caregivers and individuals living with dementia and an increase in job satisfaction for staff," according to the Alzheimer's Association. I provided you with a handout with details on some states with significantly lower median monthly costs who also require anywhere from 8 hours to 16 hours of annual continuing education specific to dementia care. Alabama, Arizona, and Wyoming are among a few states with such requirements. The median monthly cost for facilities in these states is $5,095, $6,000, and $4,025 respectively. People with dementia are a vulnerable population, requiring special care. This bill is a step towards safer, quality care for residents of facilities and a safer work environment for the staff who serve them. Let's join the states who have prioritized the need for dementia care training. We hope you support this.

Source: Delaware Title 16 Division of Health Care Quality 3225 Assisted Living Facilities, Delaware Title 16 Division of Health Care Quality 3220 Training and Qualifications for Certified Nursing Assistants, "How Much Does Memory Care Cost? A Complete State-by-State Guide" published on May 1, 2024 on A Place For Mom, Alzheimer's Association website

A bill outside of the long-term care bill package was also designed to improve oversight of staff in facilities. House Bill 204 "grants authority to the Department of Health & Social Services to adopt regulations related to the operation of temporary staffing agencies that staff temporary nurses and other staff positions in long-term care facilities." The Division of Health Care Quality will have oversight of the agencies, including staff qualifications, credentials, and job requirements. Temporary staffing agencies were becoming more common yet did not have state oversight without this bill. While my coalition and I did not comment on the first committee hearing, I spoke in support of it in the Senate Committee meeting. Based on comments during the hearing, the long-term care industry advocated for the bill, too.

HB 204- Senate Health & Social Services Committee, June 18, 2024

We were in the final stretches of the legislative session with no bills yet through the full process. There were twelve days left in the session, and committees did not meet every day. My faith had been tested, and I couldn't imagine all the effort of the last few months not resulting in at least one law. On my way driving to Dover that morning, as I was exiting the highway, a car with the license plate "HISWILL" pulled in front of me. It reminded me that I could prepare as much as possible, but I was not in control of what happens. Feeling renewed in my strength, I effectively gave my speech, and the bill moved forward through committee—one step closer to law.

I'm Candace Esham, founder of the Delaware Elder Care Advocacy Coalition. We support HB 204. With long-term care facilities increasingly relying on temporary staffing agencies, it is critical DHSS has oversight of the qualifications of all provided staff as well as other records. According to Consumer

Voice, nursing homes, on average experience turnover of 52% of nursing staff each year. This turnover can contribute to the usage of temporary staff. The article states turnover is related to poor pay, lack of benefits, high workloads, inadequate training, poor management, and lack of career advancement. Until these key factors impacting the facility workforce are addressed, the higher utilization of temporary staffing agencies will continue. This bill is a step towards safer, quality care for residents of facilities and a safer work environment for the staff who serve them, both in house and temporary.

Source: "High staff turnover: a job quality crisis in nursing homes" in *The National Consumer Voice for Quality Long-Term Care* published September 8, 2022

https://theconsumervoice.org/uploads/files/issues/High_Staff_Turnover-A_Job_Quality_Crisis_in_Nursing_Homes.pdf

---

SB 215- House Appropriations Committee, June 25, 2024

I'm Candace Esham, founder of the Delaware Elder Care Advocacy Coalition. We support SB 215.

Quality care and fiscal responsibility go hand in hand. Last year, long-term care facilities in Delaware received an extra $25 million and JFC didn't know where the money went during the meetings held in February. This year they will get an extra $7 million in state funding and $10 million in federal, bringing the total state and federal investment over the last two years to $40 million. The cost of surveys pales in comparison to this and surveys provide *oversight to these significant investments. Funding is needed for qualified surveyors, who at this time are mostly contractors. It is not only a safety matter for residents but ensures the operators of facilities enable their staff to provide better care and taxpayer dollars are invested well.*

Source: Senate Bill 195 (FY24 Budget Bill), Senate Bill 325 (FY25 Budget Bill)

By the end of June 30th, six of the bills we partnered with legislators on received unanimous support from the Senate and House. In the history of Delaware, there were never six bills passed at once in relation to long-term care facilities. Senator Mantzavinos and Representative Johnson ensured the voices of our most vulnerable were heard through families in my coalition. On August 1, 2024, Governor Carney held a signing in Wilmington, Delaware for five of the bills with key stakeholders invited. I wore a bracelet engraved with Isaiah 41:10, "do not fear for I am with you," and Memom's engagement ring. When I turned on my car to drive to the signing ceremony, "Walk On Faith" by Mike Reid was playing on the radio. While I had never heard this song before, I reflected on the importance of faith over fear in life. In the penthouse of the Carvel Building, I gathered with some members of my coalition as years of advocacy proved to make a difference. Senator Mantzavinos and Representative Johnson stated they remained committed to continuing to improve care for Delaware seniors, and this was just the beginning. Governor Carney noticed, as he was signing each bill, how rare it is to have unanimous approval. The bills combined are steps to improve oversight, accountability, and training, which will benefit residents and the workforce in long-term care facilities. Systemic issues in the care for seniors are not unique to Delaware. Modeling best practices from other states provided the platform for steps toward improving quality care. While no state has the "perfect formula" for regulations for care, it will take learning what works and aiming to continuously improve to ensure our seniors are given the opportunity to thrive. The 152nd legislative session's success energized families, including mine.

Moving forward

The legislative changes made in 2024 for seniors in long-term care facilities are just the beginning to address systemic issues in institutions. Successfully passing five bills seemed impossible at the start of the session, but as we refined our strategy and doubled down on our determination, we achieved what many thought to be impossible. After the laws are passed, the state departments develop regulations and are responsible for enforcing the laws. There will always be room to improve the complex systems that care for our seniors. However, never underestimate the power of dedicated, passionate advocates. We will continue to be a voice for those in long-term care facilities and strive to make better processes for community-based care.

Most people want to remain in their homes as they age, and the more resources provided to enable that will help reduce the number of people who believe institutionalization is the only choice. As a society, we must redesign how we view seniors and ensure our loved ones can age gracefully. Long-term care facilities are one piece of the system. Each week, I encounter someone who has either worked in a facility or knows someone in one, and they recognize drastic changes are needed. Three key strategies used to achieve success in passing six bills will continue to be valuable to drive other improvements:

1. Develop a business plan with specific objectives, ideally modeling best practices from other states or industries.
2. Build a network of allies who share the vision for a better care system and can amplify the voices of the team of advocates.
3. Always anticipate the argument from opponents to change and research the facts.

All the steps in the four years from when I started my advocacy journey to the bill signing in August 2024 were critical to influencing regulatory changes. It was difficult realizing Memom's story wouldn't be enough of a tragedy to show the problems, but once I used my professional experience in developing a business plan with statewide data, legislators could align with the goals. Residents from facilities across the nation experience neglect, and advocates for quality care need to build their network. There is power in numbers. The first major network connection in my journey was with Meredith Newman, the journalist who dedicated over 18 months to a series of articles exposing neglect and lack of oversight. Media coverage drew legislators' attention to the long-standing issues with survey frequency, complaint backlog, and harm. Approaching the discussions with not only my family's experience but with a strategy including a mission statement, goals, and research behind the recommendations proved to be beneficial. Solutions that benefit residents and the workforce showed we wanted to partner with stakeholders. This led to a powerful network of allies committed to progress over perfection. Finally, knowing the perspective of opponents to bills and exposing the data behind their position helped shine a light on how facilities in other states prioritized quality improvement programs. State and federal regulations for senior care need to be effective and transparent to ensure the best care is given. Aging with dignity is a basic human right and how we should all aspire to be treated.

Acknowledgements

Proverbs 28:1 "The wicked flee when no one
pursues, but the righteous are bold as a lion"

First, I want to thank my parents for their unwavering support and for encouraging me to share our story. They remind me I need to have faith and give me strength to keep going. I am grateful they believe I can conquer anything I decide to tackle. Kelli, Andrea, Christine, and Becca shared tears with me over the years and celebrated each step towards making changes. Kelsey connecting me with Meredith Newman, an exceptional investigative journalist who became a friend during the years of investigation, helped bring state-wide acknowledgement of the years of neglect seniors have suffered. The article featuring Memom and the systemic issues in Delaware festering for years finally garnered the attention of legislators.

Senator Mantzavinos and Representative Johnson are true leaders who did not fear the complexity of the issues preventing quality care. During the session, their peers challenged the bills, even claiming higher standards "impossible." Providing families a voice in a room full of opposition is a gift I will always cherish. As I began to document the progress of legislation, I asked a few colleagues for an early review of my book proposal. I'm appreciative of David, Janet, Mary Lib, Dr. Sleesman, and mom for their invaluable encouragement and thoughts on how to tell a clear story.

My family's experience with neglect in a long-term care facility unfortunately is not unique. In writing this book and advocating for change, I finally started to heal. Before Memom passed away, my decisions were based upon fear. I worried reporting issues would result in retaliation, choices made would cause more harm, or even speaking up about isolation would cause backlash against me. Once I decided to develop a strategy with my coalition and develop solutions, there was a shift in how I carried my grief. In this book, I did not describe the physical, mental, and emotional toll of the last few years and how it impacted my health. This was not to minimize the reality, but I did not want to distract from the bigger picture of senior neglect. My wellness team including Dr. Doshi, Dr. Rob, Terry, Ciera, Frank, and Joe helped me get to the root causes of my pain and gave me the tools to be able to have energy to advocate and write. I plan to explain the health issues in another story.

To my publisher, Defiance Press & Publishing, thank you for believing in the importance of my story and giving me a platform to help others. On the evening that I signed the contract with my publisher, I saw a license plate that said, "Ask God." One more sign to keep spreading light and never lose faith. Finally, to my fellow Delaware Elder Care Advocacy Coalition members, I am sorry we are bonded by tragedy, but I am forever grateful for your unwavering strength. Thank you for believing in each other, especially in me, and honoring your loved ones as we strive for improvements. Here's to never giving up hope.

www.ingramcontent.com/pod-product-compliance
Lightning Source LLC
Chambersburg PA
CBHW062216270326
41930CB00009B/1752